# MACRO
## *Cookbook*
# FOR BEGINNERS

A Comprehensive Beginner's Guide to Crafting
Delicious and Nutrient-Dense Macro Meals

JOSELYN CLARK

# CONTENTS

# INTRODUCTION

Welcome to the Macro Cookbook for Beginners! If you've ever been curious about macro-counting, looking to make informed dietary choices, or want to gain a better understanding of your food, this book is for you.

**Newcomers to Macro Nutrition:** This book is created for those new to macro-nutrients who want to delve into macro counting and mindful eating. If you've never tracked your macros or aren't sure where to start, you're in the right place.

**Health Enthusiasts:** If you're passionate about your health and wellness, this cookbook allows you to fine-tune your nutritional approach. Understanding macros empowers you to make more informed choices about your foods.

**Fitness Enthusiasts:** Whether you're an athlete, a weekend warrior, or simply someone who enjoys regular physical activity, the Macro Cookbook for Beginners will help you optimize your nutrition to support your fitness goals.

**Weight Management Seekers:** Macros can be a powerful tool if you're working toward weight loss or weight maintenance. This book offers insights into balancing your macronutrient intake to meet your goals.

**Anyone Seeking Dietary Knowledge:** This book provides an educational foundation for those who want to cultivate a deeper connection with their food and better understand how different nutrients impact their bodies.

The Macro Cookbook for Beginners is your gateway to macro nutrition. We created this book to provide a comprehensive, beginner-friendly resource to understand, track, and optimize your macronutrient intake.

**1. Simplicity for Starters:** Macros can seem overwhelming, but we've designed this cookbook with beginners in mind. We break down the fundamentals of macronutrients clearly and straightforwardly.

**2. Practical Guidance:** You'll find practical tips, meal planning strategies, and beginner-friendly recipes that make macro counting and mindful eating accessible and enjoyable.

**3. A Holistic Approach:** Our book goes beyond just numbers; it encourages you to consider the quality of the foods you consume. We emphasize the importance of whole, nutrient-dense ingredients.

**4. Recipe Variety:** The Macro Cookbook for Beginners isn't just about theory; it's packed with a wide range of delicious recipes, from breakfast to dinner, to ensure you enjoy every bite.

**5. Empowerment:** By understanding macros, you gain the power to make informed choices about your diet. This knowledge can be a game-changer for your health, fitness, and overall well-being.

The Macro Cookbook for Beginners is your starting point in exploring the world of macro nutrition. Whether you're here to gain insight into your diet, improve your health, enhance your fitness journey, or enjoy flavorful meals, we're excited to be your guide. Your macro adventure begins here!

# Chapter 1

# Macros and the Macro Diet Explained

Before you dive into the recipes and meal plans in the Macro Cookbook for Beginners, it's crucial to understand the foundation of this dietary approach.

## What Are Macros?

"Macros" is short for macronutrients, the three primary nutrients that make up the caloric content of our foods. These macronutrients are:

**1. Carbohydrates (Carbs):** Carbohydrates are the body's primary energy source. They consist of sugars, starches, and fiber. They are contained in various foods, from grains and fruits to vegetables and legumes.

**2. Proteins:** Proteins are essential for the repair and growth of tissues in your body. They're made up of amino acids and can be found in foods like meat, poultry, fish, beans, and dairy products.

**3. Fats:** Fats are another energy source and serve various bodily functions, helping absorb fat-soluble vitamins. They come in different forms, such as saturated, unsaturated, and trans fats. They are in foods like avocados, nuts, oils, and butter.

## The Significance of Macros

Understanding macros is crucial because they are fundamental to how your body functions. Here's a closer look at why macros matter:

**Energy:** Carbohydrates and fats are the body's primary energy sources. They fuel your daily activities and bodily functions. Consuming the right balance of these macros ensures you have enough energy to power through your day.

**Muscle Health:** Proteins are the building blocks of muscles and tissues. If you're aiming to build or maintain strength, protein is essential. It also plays a role in enzyme and hormone production.

**Hormone Regulation:** Fats, specifically essential fatty acids, are integral to hormone production and regulation in the body. Hormones control various processes, including metabolism, mood, and growth.

**Satiety:** Different macros affect your fullness and satisfaction after a meal. Balancing your macros can help you manage hunger and prevent overeating.

## Understanding Macro Ratios

A fundamental principle in macro nutrition is the balance of these three macronutrients in your diet. This balance is often expressed as a ratio, with the most common being:

- 40% Carbohydrates, 30% Protein, 30% Fat: A balanced approach.
- 50% Carbohydrates, 20% Protein, 30% Fat: Common for endurance athletes.
- 30% Carbohydrates, 40% Protein, 30% Fat: Preferred by some bodybuilders.

Your proper ratio depends on your goals, activity level, and dietary preferences. By tracking your macros, you can tailor your diet to suit your needs, whether focused on weight loss, muscle gain, or overall well-being.

## Macro Counting

Macro counting tracks the grams of carbohydrates, proteins, and fats you consume daily to meet your macro ratio. This process can be done using food scales, nutrition apps, or consulting a nutritionist.

By understanding macros and tracking them, you can gain precise control over your diet, making it a versatile and practical approach to achieving your nutritional and health goals.

As you start your journey into the Macro Cookbook for Beginners, remember that macros are the building blocks of your diet. They influence your energy levels, muscle health, and hormone regulation. By understanding macro principles and counting your macros, you gain the power to tailor your nutrition to your unique goals and preferences. This knowledge is the foundation we'll build in the following chapters, where you'll explore delicious and balanced recipes that align with your macro goals.

# The Crucial Role of Macros in Your Diet

In the Macro Cookbook for Beginners, we've already introduced you to the world of macronutrients and their significance. Now, let's delve deeper into the importance of macros and how they impact your diet, health, and overall well-being.

### 1. Energy Source: Fueling Your Body

Macronutrients are your body's primary source of energy. Carbohydrates and fats are like the gasoline in your body's engine, powering all your daily activities, from the simplest tasks to the most complex processes. You may feel sluggish and tired without an adequate balance of carbs and fats.

- **Carbohydrates:** These fast-acting energy sources are essential for high-intensity activities and brain function. They are rapidly converted into glucose, which fuels your cells.
- **Fats:** Fats are the slow-release energy sources. They provide a steady supply of energy over a more extended period. They are crucial for endurance activities and overall body functions.

Maintaining the right balance of these macros ensures your body has a constant supply of energy to function optimally.

### 2. Building and Repair: The Role of Proteins

Proteins, the third macronutrient, are essential for repairing, growing, and maintaining tissues in your body. They comprise amino acids, which serve as the building blocks for various structures, including muscles, skin, hair, and enzymes. Here's how proteins play a crucial role:

- **Muscle Health:** For those in fitness, adequate protein intake is essential to support muscle growth and repair. Even if you're not an athlete, your muscles require protein for maintenance and repair.
- **Tissue Regeneration:** Beyond muscles, proteins are involved in tissue repair and regeneration, ensuring you remain healthy and strong.

### 3. Hormone Regulation: Maintaining Balance

Fats, specifically essential fatty acids, are integral to hormone production and regulation. Hormones are the body's messengers, controlling various processes, including metabolism, mood, and growth. When your fat intake is too low or imbalanced, it can disrupt your hormone regulation, potentially leading to health issues.

For example, omega-3 and omega-6 fatty acids are crucial for brain health and mood regulation. Without an adequate supply of these essential fats, you might experience mood swings, poor concentration, or even depressive symptoms.

### 4. Satiety: Managing Hunger

Different macros affect your feelings of fullness and satisfaction after a meal. Balancing your macros can help you manage hunger and prevent overeating. Here's how it works:

- **Carbohydrates** are typically fast-digesting and can cause rapid spikes and crashes in blood sugar levels. By pairing carbs with proteins and fats, you can experience more stable energy and appetite control.
- **Proteins and Fats:** These macronutrients are known for promoting feelings of fullness. You can curb your appetite and avoid excessive snacking by consuming adequate proteins and healthy fats.

Understanding the importance of macros in your diet is like having a blueprint for your health. Macros provide:

- The energy to fuel your activities.
- The building blocks for your body's structures.
- The messengers that maintain balance within you.

By striking the right balance of carbohydrates, proteins, and fats, you're setting yourself on a path to health, vitality, and a well-functioning body. In the following chapters, you'll explore how to apply this knowledge in your everyday meals, creating delicious dishes that align with your macro goals.

# Building a Balanced Macro Meal with Ease

In the Macro Cookbook for Beginners, we're committed to helping you understand and apply the principles of macro nutrition in your daily life. This chapter is your practical guide to crafting well-balanced meals that align with your macro goals, promoting health and well-being.

## Building Blocks of a Balanced Macro Meal

Now, let's explore how to create a balanced macro meal:

**1. Start with Protein:** Begin by selecting your protein source. This could be lean meat, poultry, fish, tofu, legumes, or dairy products. Proteins typically comprise around 20-40% of your meal, depending on your macro ratio.

**2. Add Carbohydrates:** Next, incorporate carbohydrates, such as whole grains, fruits, or vegetables. Carbs should generally account for 40-50% of your meal, but this can vary based on your goals and activity level.

**3. Include Healthy Fats:** Finally, include sources of healthy fats in your meal, like avocados, nuts, seeds, or olive oil. Fats typically make up around 20-30% of your feed, but this, too, can be adjusted based on your specific needs.

## Portion Control

To maintain your macro ratios accurately, you may need to weigh or measure your portions, especially when starting with macro nutrition. Food scales and measuring cups can be valuable tools for ensuring you're on track. As you become more comfortable with macro counting, you may rely less on these tools.

## Balancing Your Macros for Different Meals

Each meal you consume should align with your overall daily macro ratio. However, your needs can vary depending on your activity level and timing. For instance:

- **Pre-workout:** Prioritize a carb-protein combo for energy.
- **Post-workout:** Include protein to aid muscle recovery.
- **Evening meal:** Balance your macros for a more even energy supply.

## Meal Planning

To create a balanced macro meal, consider meal planning. It can help you prepare balanced meals in advance, ensuring you consistently meet your macro goals. Additionally, meal planning can save time and quickly reduce the temptation to opt for less healthy options.

Balancing your macros may seem complex, but it becomes second nature with practice. You can create meals that align with your health and fitness goals by understanding your macro ratio, selecting appropriate foods, and paying attention to portion control. The Macro Cookbook for Beginners offers a variety of recipes to inspire and guide you on your journey to delicious, balanced macro meals. Whether you're seeking weight management, muscle gain, or better health, the key is in your hands – and on your plate.

# Allowed and Prohibited Ingredients for Your Macro Journey

As you dive deeper into the Macro Cookbook for Beginners, you must know the ingredients that can help or hinder your macro goals. This chapter will explore which components are allowed and best avoided on your macro journey.

## Allowed Ingredients

- **Lean Protein Sources:** Choose from an array of lean protein sources like skinless poultry, lean cuts of beef or pork, fish, tofu, and legumes. These are the building blocks of muscle and a great way to meet your protein goals.
- **Whole Grains:** Incorporate whole grains such as brown rice, quinoa, whole wheat pasta, and oats. These are excellent sources of complex carbohydrates that provide sustained energy.
- **Colorful Vegetables:** Embrace a variety of colorful vegetables like spinach, broccoli, bell peppers, and carrots. They're rich in vitamins, minerals, and fiber, making them perfect for meals.
- **Fruits:** Enjoy a wide selection of fruits, from berries to apples and citrus fruits. While some fruits are higher in sugar, they can still be part of a balanced diet when consumed in moderation.
- **Healthy Fats:** Include healthy fats like avocados, nuts, seeds, and olive oil. These provide essential fatty acids that support overall health.
- **Dairy and Dairy Alternatives:** Low-fat dairy products or dairy alternatives like almond milk and Greek yogurt can be part of your macro-friendly meals, offering a source of protein and calcium.
- **Herbs and Spices:** Enhance your meals with various herbs and spices. They add flavor without significant macronutrient content, making them valuable to your dishes.

## Prohibited Ingredients

- **Trans Fats:** Avoid trans fats, often found in processed and fried foods. These fats can be detrimental to your health and should be kept to a minimum or eliminated.
- **Added Sugars:** Excessive added sugars, present in sugary snacks, sugary drinks, and some cereals, can sabotage your macro goals. Limit your sugar intake as much as possible.
- **Highly Processed Foods:** Highly processed foods are often high in empty calories and low in nutrients. They can make it challenging to meet your macro goals, so it's best to minimize their consumption.
- **Sugary Beverages:** Sodas, energy drinks, and many fruit juices can be high in added sugars. Opt for water, herbal tea, or other low-calorie beverages to stay hydrated.
- **Excessively Fatty Cuts of Meat:** While proteins are essential, it's wise to choose lean cuts of meat to avoid excessive fat intake. Fatty meats can be high in unhealthy saturated fats.
- **Alcohol:** Alcohol can be high in empty calories and can affect your ability to make healthy food choices. Consuming in moderation can be part of a balanced diet, but excessive consumption should be avoided.
- **Refined Grains:** Refined grains, such as white bread and sugary cereals, have stripped their fiber and nutrients away. These can lead to rapid blood sugar spikes and are best limited.

Knowing which ingredients to include and which to avoid is a crucial aspect of macro nutrition. By selecting foods from the list of allowed ingredients and minimizing or eliminating those in the prohibited category, you'll be better equipped to meet your macro goals and maintain a balanced and healthy diet. In the upcoming chapters, you'll find many delicious recipes that showcase these ingredients, helping you craft meals that align with your macro journey.

# Proteins for a Macro-Focused Diet: Exploring Different Sources and Calculating Your Requirements

In the world of macro nutrition, proteins hold a special place. They are the building blocks for muscle, aid in tissue repair, and are essential to a balanced diet. This chapter delves into different protein sources and guides you in calculating your protein requirements for a successful macro-focused diet.

## Diverse Protein Sources

Variety in protein sources makes your meals more exciting and ensures you receive a broad spectrum of nutrients. Here are some familiar sources of protein to consider for your macro-focused diet:

1. **Lean Meats:** Skinless poultry, lean cuts of beef, pork, and game meats are excellent choices. They are low in fat and protein, making them staples in many macro-friendly diets.
2. **Fish:** Fish, particularly salmon, trout, and mackerel, are not only rich in protein but also provide valuable omega-3 fatty acids, which promote heart and brain health.
3. **Tofu and Tempeh:** These soy-based products are perfect for vegetarians and vegans. They offer a complete source of plant-based protein.
4. **Legumes:** Beans, lentils, and chickpeas are not only high in protein but also rich in fiber. They are an excellent addition to vegetarian and vegan diets.
5. **Dairy Products:** Greek yogurt, cottage cheese, and low-fat milk are good protein sources. Greek yogurt, in particular, is a favorite for its creamy texture and versatility.
6. **Eggs:** Eggs are a complete protein source and can be prepared in numerous ways, making them a versatile ingredient for your meals.
7. **Protein Supplements:** Protein supplements like whey or plant-based protein powders can be convenient for meeting your protein goals, especially if you're on the go or following a specific dietary regimen.

## Calculating Your Protein Requirements

Calculating your daily protein requirements is important in creating a macro-focused diet tailored to your needs. Here's a simplified guide to help you determine your protein needs:

1. **Determine Your Activity Level:** The more active you are, the more protein you require. For a passive person, aim for around 0.36 grams of protein per pound of body weight. Consider 0.5 to 0.7 grams per pound for those engaging in regular exercise.
2. **Set Your Goals:** Your protein intake can vary depending on your goals. Aim for the higher range if you're focused on muscle-building or intense training. Stay within the lower back if you're trying to maintain your current physique or follow a balanced diet.
3. **Do the Math:** Multiply your body weight (in pounds) by the recommended protein intake per pound to calculate your daily protein requirement. For example, if you weigh 150 pounds and are moderately active, you might aim for 75-105 grams of protein daily.

Proteins are the puzzle pieces that help your body function optimally. They support muscle growth, aid in tissue repair, and keep you feeling full and satisfied. By diversifying your protein sources and calculating your requirements, you can harness the power of proteins to achieve your macro nutrition goals.

# Carbohydrates: Fueling Your Body with Purpose

Carbohydrates often need to be understood in the world of nutrition. In this chapter of the Macro Cookbook for Beginners, we'll uncover carbohydrates' critical role in fueling your body and explore the diverse, healthy sources of carbs that can become your dietary allies.

## Understanding the Role of Carbohydrates

Carbohydrates are your body's primary source of energy, and they play several crucial roles in your overall health:

- **Energy Production:** Carbs are efficiently converted into glucose, providing a quick energy source that fuels your everyday activities, from taking a stroll to completing a strenuous workout.
- **Brain Function:** Glucose from carbs is essential for brain function. It enhances cognitive performance, supports memory, and improves concentration.
- **Muscle Energy:** During high-intensity exercise, your muscles rely on carbohydrates to perform optimally. Carbs are stored as glycogen in muscles and tapped into for power bursts.
- **Digestive Health:** Carbohydrates, particularly those from whole grains, fruits, and vegetables, are rich in dietary fiber. Fiber promotes healthy digestion, helps maintain regular bowel movements, and may lower the risk of chronic diseases.

## Healthy Sources of Carbs

Not all carbohydrates are created equal. The key is to focus on healthy sources that provide essential nutrients and fiber. Here are some carbohydrate-rich foods to incorporate into your macro-focused diet:

1. **Whole Grains:** Whole grains like brown rice, quinoa, whole wheat pasta, and oats are packed with complex carbohydrates, fiber, vitamins, and minerals.
2. **Legumes:** Beans, lentils, and chickpeas are excellent sources of carbs and provide a healthy dose of plant-based protein and fiber.
3. **Fruits:** Fruits such as apples, berries, oranges, and bananas offer natural sugars, fiber, and an array of vitamins.
4. **Vegetables:** Leafy greens, broccoli, carrots, and bell peppers are just a few examples of vegetables rich in carbohydrates, fiber, and essential nutrients.
5. **Sweet Potatoes:** These starchy vegetables provide healthy carbs, vitamins, and minerals. They're a great addition to your meals, offering sustained energy.
6. **Dairy:** Low-fat dairy products like yogurt and milk contain natural sugars, making them a good carbohydrate source that also offers calcium and protein.
7. **Nuts and Seeds:** Nuts and seeds like almonds, chia seeds, and flaxseeds are carbohydrate-rich and provide healthy fats, protein, and fiber.

## Balancing Your Carbs

Balancing your carbohydrate intake is essential for achieving your macro goals. The key is to choose nutrient-dense, complex carbohydrates over refined and simple sugars. This approach helps you meet your daily energy needs and provides essential vitamins and minerals to support overall health.

Carbohydrates are your body's primary fuel source, powering everything from your morning jog to your afternoon brainstorming session. By selecting healthy sources of carbs rich in nutrients and fiber, you can harness their energy-boosting potential while promoting your overall well-being.

# Fats: Essential for Macros and Health

In the Macro Cookbook for Beginners, fats often take a back seat to carbohydrates and proteins. However, fats are crucial for your macros and overall health.

## The Truth About Dietary Fats

Fats are often misunderstood, and their reputation has been tarnished. It's important to recognize that fats are essential nutrients with numerous vital functions in the body:

1. **Energy Storage:** Fats are your body's primary long-term energy storage. They provide a consistent source of fuel during periods of low food intake.
2. **Cellular Structure:** Fats are essential components of cell membranes and play a critical role in maintaining the integrity and functionality of your cells.
3. **Nutrient Absorption:** Some vitamins, like A, D, E, and K, are fat-soluble, which means they need fats for proper absorption.
4. **Brain Health:** Fats, particularly omega-3 fatty acids, are crucial for brain health, supporting cognitive function and mood regulation.

## Healthy Fats vs. Unhealthy Fats

Not all fats are created equal, and distinguishing between healthy and unhealthy fats is critical to making intelligent dietary choices:

**Healthy Fats:**

1. **Monounsaturated Fats:** These fats are found in olive oil, avocados, and nuts. They have been linked to heart health and may help reduce harmful cholesterol levels.
2. **Polyunsaturated Fats:** Omega-3 and Omega-6 fatty acids fall into this category. They support brain function, reduce inflammation, and offer numerous health benefits. Fatty fish like salmon, flaxseeds, and walnuts are rich sources.

**Unhealthy Fats:**

1. **Saturated** fats are primarily found in animal products like meat and dairy and some tropical oils like coconut and palm oil. Consuming too much-saturated fats can raise harmful cholesterol levels and increase the risk of heart disease.
2. **Trans Fats:** Trans fats are primarily artificial fats created through hydrogenation, turning liquid oils into solid fats. Trans fats are found in many processed and fried foods and are considered highly unhealthy.

## Incorporating Fats into Your Diet

Balancing your fat intake within your macro-focused diet is essential for overall health and achieving your nutritional goals. Here's how you can incorporate healthy fats into your meals:

1. **Cooking Oils:** Opt for olive, avocado, or canola oil. These oils are rich in monounsaturated fats and offer a pleasant dish flavor.
2. **Avocados:** Avocado is a versatile fruit that can be added to salads, sandwiches, or creamy dips and dressings.
3. **Fatty Fish:** Include fatty fish like salmon, mackerel, and trout at least twice a week. These fish provide both healthy fats and high-quality protein.
4. **Nuts and Seeds:** Incorporate nuts and seeds, such as almonds, walnuts, flaxseeds, and chia seeds, into your meals or enjoy them as a snack.
5. **Nut Butters:** Nut butters like almond or peanut butter are delicious spreads used in sandwiches, oatmeal, or as a dip for fruit.
6. **Dairy Products:** Opt for low-fat dairy products like yogurt, milk, and cheese to obtain healthy fats and essential nutrients like calcium and protein.

Fats may be the unsung heroes of your macro nutrition journey. They are essential for energy storage, cellular health, nutrient absorption, and well-being. By embracing healthy fats and limiting unhealthy fats, you can enhance your health while fine-tuning your macros.



# Chapter 2

# Making the Macro Diet Work for You

In the Macro Cookbook for Beginners, we've explored the intricacies of macronutrients, their sources, and their significance. Now, let's discuss how to make the macro diet work for you in practical terms.

## Cooking and Preparing Macros

To master the macro diet, becoming skilled in cooking and meal preparation is essential. Here's how to do it right:

1. **Meal Planning:** Plan your meals to align with your macro goals. This can save time, reduce the likelihood of unhealthy choices, and streamline your cooking process.
2. **Food Scale:** Invest in a reliable food scale. Weighing your ingredients helps you accurately track your macros, ensuring you stay on target.
3. **Smart Shopping:** Purchase fresh, whole ingredients rich in proteins, healthy carbs, and good fats. Shopping for the right foods is the first step to creating balanced meals.
4. **Batch Cooking:** Cook in batches to save time and effort. Prepare more significant portions and store them in the refrigerator or freezer for future meals.
5. **Kitchen Tools:** Equip your kitchen with essential tools like measuring cups, quality knives, and versatile cookware. These make the cooking process more efficient.

## Cooking Techniques for Balanced Macros

Cooking your macros requires understanding the cooking techniques that help you create balanced meals. Here are some methods to keep in mind:

1. **Grilling:** Grilling is a healthy way to cook proteins and vegetables. It adds flavor without unnecessary fats.
2. **Stir-Frying:** Stir-frying is a quick and efficient way to prepare balanced meals, allowing you to incorporate lean proteins, colorful veggies, and healthy fats.
3. **Baking:** Baking is a versatile method for preparing proteins, vegetables, and whole grains like quinoa. It retains nutrients and flavors.
4. **Steaming:** Steaming is an excellent technique for preserving the nutritional value of vegetables. It's quick and maintains the crunch and color of your veggies.
5. **Sautéing:** Sautéing with olive oil or other healthy fats enhances the flavors of your ingredients. It's excellent for cooking proteins, vegetables, or whole grains.

## Tips for Beginners in Macro Tracking

Macro tracking can initially seem daunting, but it becomes a natural part of your dietary routine with practice. Here are some tips for beginners:

1. **Use Apps:** Utilize macro tracking apps to make the process more accessible. These apps allow you to scan barcodes, input recipes, and calculate macros effortlessly.
2. **Plan Ahead:** Plan your meals to ensure your macros align with your goals. This reduces last-minute, uncalculated decisions.
3. **Keep It Simple:** Start with simple meals and gradually expand your culinary horizons. Simple recipes are more accessible to track and manage.

4. **Be Patient:** Learning to track macros takes time. Don't be discouraged by early challenges; persistence is vital to success.

5. **Seek Support:** Share your journey with friends or seek support from online communities. Others' experiences and advice can be invaluable.

You must become proficient in cooking and meal preparation to make the macro diet work. This chapter has introduced you to fundamental techniques and tips for tracking macros efficiently and effectively. As you continue your journey through the Macro Cookbook for Beginners, you'll gain practical experience in preparing delicious, balanced meals that align with your macro goals. It's all about making this nutritional approach a sustainable and enjoyable part of your lifestyle.

# Macros and Specific Dietary Needs

In the Macro Cookbook for Beginners, we've delved into the essential concepts of macronutrients and how to craft a balanced macro-focused diet. However, we understand that dietary preferences and restrictions often play a significant role in your food choices.

## Understanding Specific Dietary Needs

Different dietary needs arise from various factors, including health considerations, ethical choices, allergies, and personal preferences. Here are some specific nutritional deficiencies you might encounter:

1. **Vegan:** A vegan diet eliminates all animal products, including meat, dairy, eggs, and honey. Plant-based protein sources are essential for vegans.

2. **Vegetarian:** Vegetarians abstain from meat but may consume dairy and eggs. Ensuring an adequate protein intake, particularly for lacto-ovo vegetarians, is essential.

3. **Gluten-Free:** Gluten is found in wheat, barley, and rye. Those with celiac disease or gluten sensitivity need to avoid these grains. Gluten-free grains like rice, quinoa, and corn can be part of their diet.

4. **Lactose-Free:** Lactose intolerance can make dairy consumption challenging. Lactose-free dairy or dairy alternatives like almond milk can be suitable.

5. **Pescatarian:** Pescatarians consume fish and seafood but avoid other meats. They often focus on lean proteins and omega-3-rich fish.

6. **Low-Carb/Keto:** Low-carb and keto diets emphasize minimal carbohydrate intake and rely heavily on fats and proteins for energy.

7. **Paleo:** The paleo diet centers on whole foods similar to what our ancestors might have eaten, focusing on lean meats, fish, fruits, vegetables, nuts, and seeds while avoiding processed foods and grains.

## Adapting the Macro Diet to Specific Dietary Needs

Adapting your macro-focused diet to specific dietary needs can be straightforward and rewarding. Here's how:

1. **Select the Right Proteins:** Depending on your dietary needs, choose plant-based proteins, dairy or dairy alternatives, fish, or lean meats. Tofu, tempeh, and legumes are excellent choices for vegans and vegetarians.

2. **Choose Carbohydrate Sources Wisely:** Choose carbohydrates that align with your dietary restrictions. For gluten-free diets, focus on gluten-free grains like rice or quinoa. Replace starchy carbs with non-starchy vegetables and nuts for low-carb or keto diets.

3. **Healthy Fats:** Healthy fats like avocados, nuts, and olive oil suit most dietary needs. However, ensure they fit your specific dietary restrictions.

4. **Supplements:** Some dietary needs may require supplementation. For example,

vegans often need to supplement with vitamin B12 and iron.

5. **Recipe Adaptations:** Modify recipes to meet your specific dietary requirements. Replace animal proteins with plant-based alternatives or adapt recipes to avoid gluten or dairy.

The beauty of the macro diet is its adaptability. Regardless of your dietary needs, you can tailor your macro-focused diet to meet your goals and restrictions. This chapter has provided insight into navigating various dietary preferences and requirements, ensuring that the macro diet is accessible and enjoyable for everyone, regardless of their unique needs.

# Tailoring Macros for Special Diets

In the Macro Cookbook for Beginners, we've explored the versatility of macronutrients and how to incorporate them into various dietary needs. Now, we'll delve even deeper into the art of tailoring macros for special diets.

## Understanding Special Diets

Special diets often serve specific purposes, whether it's weight loss, managing a medical condition, or optimizing athletic performance. Here are some special diets that may require macro tailoring:

1. **Ketogenic Diet:** The keto diet is an ultra-low-carb, high-fat diet that forces your body into ketosis, burning fat for energy. Macros typically comprise 70-75% fat, 20-25% protein, and 5-10% carbohydrates.

2. **Low-Carb Diet:** Low-carb diets restrict carb intake to promote weight loss or blood sugar control. Macros often include around 20-50% carbohydrates, with the rest coming from protein and fat.

3. **High-Protein Diet:** High-protein diets emphasize protein intake to support muscle growth and weight loss. Macros may consist of 30-40% protein, 30-40% carbohydrates, and 20-30% fat.

4. **Intermittent Fasting:** Intermittent fasting focuses on when you eat rather than what you eat. Macros are consumed during specific time windows.

5. **Bodybuilder Diet:** Bodybuilders often adopt a high-protein, moderate-carb, low-fat diet. Macros could be around 40% protein, 40% carbohydrates, and 20% fat.

## Tailoring Macros for Special Diets

Adapting your macros for special diets is both a science and an art. Here's how to tailor your macro-focused diet to specific dietary requirements:

**Ketogenic Diet:** For keto, focus on reducing carbs to minimal levels, emphasizing fats and moderating protein. Foods like avocados, nuts, olive oil, and fatty fish should become dietary staples.

**Low-Carb Diet:** Keep carb intake within the specified range for a low-carb diet. Substitute starchy carbs with non-starchy vegetables and select lean proteins and healthy fats.

**High-Protein Diet:** On a high-protein diet, protein-rich foods become the star. To meet your protein goals, include lean meats, poultry, fish, legumes, and tofu.

**Intermittent Fasting:** During intermittent fasting, adjust your macros to fit your eating window. Ensure you consume the necessary nutrients within your designated time frame.

**Bodybuilder Diet:** On a bodybuilder's diet, prioritize lean proteins, complex carbohydrates, and minimal fats. Make use of whole grains, poultry, lean meats, and vegetables.

## Recipe Adaptations for Special Diets

Modify recipes to meet your specific dietary needs. Replace or adjust ingredients to fit your macros and preferences. Special diets may call for creative and tasty adaptations that align with your goals and restrictions.

Special diets offer a personalized approach to nutrition, allowing you to address specific goals or health needs. By understanding the principles of macro tailoring, you can make the macro diet work for you, regardless of your unique requirements.

# Eating Out and Macros

Eating out is a delightful way to experience new flavors and cuisines. Still, it can present challenges when sticking to your macro-focused diet.

## Dining at Restaurants and Tracking Macros

Whether it's a cozy local café or a fine dining establishment, dining at restaurants is an opportunity to explore a world of flavors. To ensure you don't deviate from your macros, consider the following strategies:

1. **Plan Ahead:** Many restaurants post their menus online. Before you go, review the menu and select options that match your macro goals. Planning reduces impulsive, high-calorie choices.
2. **Watch Portions:** Restaurant portions are often more significant than you'd serve at home. When your meal arrives, consider splitting it or immediately packing half for later.
3. **Customize Your Order:** Don't hesitate to ask your server for modifications. Requesting steamed vegetables instead of fries, a lean protein option, or dressing on the side can help you control your macros.
4. **Avoid Liquid Calories:** Beverages like soda, sweetened tea, and alcoholic drinks can add significant extra calories. Stick to water, unsweetened tea, or other low-calorie options.
5. **Be Mindful of Sauces:** Many restaurant dishes come drenched in rich, calorie-dense sauces. Ask for sauces on the side or opt for lighter alternatives like vinaigrettes.
6. **Dessert Decisions:** Consider sharing with others at your table if you're craving dessert. Savoring a few bites can satisfy your sweet tooth without blowing your macros.

## Making Wise Choices When Eating Out

Making wise choices at restaurants is essential for staying on track with your macros and enjoying your dining experience. Here's how to make intelligent decisions:

1. **Lean Proteins:** Opt for dishes featuring lean proteins like grilled chicken, turkey, or fish. These options are protein-packed and lower in fats.
2. **Salads with Caution:** Salads can be both healthy and deceiving. Pay attention to toppings and dressings, as they can quickly turn a healthy salad into a calorie bomb.
3. **Steamed or Grilled:** Look for steamed, grilled, or baked dishes. These preparation methods generally add fewer calories compared to fried or sautéed options.
4. **Whole Grains:** If you have the choice, select entire grains like brown rice or quinoa instead of refined grains. They offer more nutrients and fiber.
5. **Veggies as Sides:** Opt for vegetable sides or request them instead of high-calorie sides like fries or mashed potatoes.
6. **Mindful Snacking:** If your meal is delayed, keep your appetite healthy with a basket of bread or chips. Save your macros for the main course.
7. **Stay Hydrated:** Drinking water before and during your meal can help you feel full, preventing overindulgence.

Eating out and tracking macros is a challenge. Still, enjoying restaurant dining while meeting your dietary goals is entirely possible. By planning, making wise choices, and customizing your orders, you can relish restaurants' culinary experiences while maintaining a balanced macro diet.

Navigating Fast Food and Macros

Fast food restaurants are known for their convenience but notorious for their potential to derail your macro-focused diet.

Staying Consistent with Macros

Fast food may seem like the nemesis of a macro diet, but with the right approach, it can still fit into your nutritional plan. Here's how to stay consistent with your macros when faced with fast food options:

1. **Check Nutritional Information:** Most fast food chains provide detailed nutritional information online or in restaurants. Review this information before ordering to make informed choices.
2. **Set Limits:** Establish a clear limit for your fast food meal's macros. This helps you avoid overindulgence and stay within your daily macro targets.
3. **Choose Lean Proteins:** Opt for menu items that feature lean proteins like grilled chicken, turkey, or fish. These are generally lower in fats and fit well with a macro-focused diet.
4. **Beware of Hidden Fats:** Fast food items often contain hidden fats, such as mayonnaise or cheese. Ask for these items on the side or omitted.
5. **Manage Portions:** Fast food portions are often more significant than recommended. Consider ordering a kid's meal or sharing with a friend to control your portion sizes.
6. **Skip Sugary Beverages:** Avoid sugary sodas and drink water, unsweetened tea, or diet beverages. Liquid calories can quickly add up.

Tracking Progress

Tracking your progress is a fundamental aspect of the macro diet. Here's how to do it effectively when incorporating fast food:

1. **Use Mobile Apps:** Many fast food chains have mobile apps that provide easy access to nutritional information. Use these apps to calculate your macros on the go.
2. **Keep a Food Diary:** Keep a food diary if you're away from a computer or smartphone. Write down what you eat at the fast food restaurant and calculate your macros later.
3. **Plan Ahead:** Plan your fast food choices. If you know, you'll be eating fast food, you can adjust your other meals throughout the day to accommodate it.
4. **Account for Condiments:** Remember to factor in condiments, sauces, and toppings when tracking your macros. These extras can significantly impact your calorie and macro counts.
5. **Monitor Progress:** Regularly assess your progress to ensure you're on track with your macro goals. Adjust your fast food choices and portions if necessary.

Navigating fast food while maintaining macros is feasible with some planning and self-control. By utilizing nutritional information, setting limits, and making wise choices, you can enjoy the occasional fast food meal while staying consistent with your dietary goals.

# Helpful Tools and Resources for Macro Beginners

Embarking on a journey into the world of macros as a beginner is exciting, but it can be overwhelming. In this chapter of the Macro Cookbook for Beginners, we'll introduce you to various helpful tools and resources to make your macro diet experience more accessible and enjoyable.

1. Food Scale

A reliable food scale is one of the most critical tools for tracking macros. This device helps you accurately measure and weigh your food, ensuring you stay on target with your macro goals. Invest in a digital scale with a tare function for ease of use.

## 2. Nutrition Tracking Apps

Nutrition tracking apps like MyFitnessPal, Cronometer, and Lose It! are invaluable resources for beginners. These apps offer extensive databases of foods, allowing you to log your daily intake, track your macros, and monitor your progress effortlessly. Some even allow barcode scanning for precise entries.

## 3. Online Macro Calculators

Various websites and apps offer free macro calculators. By inputting your age, weight, activity level, and goals, these calculators can help you determine your daily macro targets. They're an excellent starting point for macro beginners.

## 4. Recipe Websites and Apps

Recipe websites and apps like AllRecipes, Food Network, and Yummly offer many recipes for every dietary preference. Use these platforms to find inspiration and adapt recipes to align with your macro goals.

## 5. Kitchen Tools

Equipping your kitchen with essential tools can make macro cooking and meal preparation more accessible. Ensure you have measuring cups, spoons, a food processor, and quality cookware. Having the right tools on hand streamlines your cooking experience.

## 6. Online Communities

Online communities and forums dedicated to macros, such as Reddit's r/MealPrepSunday and various Facebook groups, can provide support and guidance. Sharing your journey and experiences with like-minded individuals can be motivating and educational.

## 7. Cookbooks

Macro-focused cookbooks can be indispensable. They provide recipes tailored to macro ratios and dietary goals, offering culinary inspiration.

## 8. Meal Planning Apps

Meal planning apps like Plan to Eat or Paprika can assist you in organizing your weekly meals, making your macro tracking routine more straightforward.

## 9. Nutrition Labels

Become familiar with reading nutrition labels on packaged foods. They provide detailed information about the macronutrient content per serving, making choosing foods that align with your goals easier.

## 10. Professional Guidance

Consider consulting a registered dietitian or nutritionist for personalized guidance. They can help you develop a macro plan that meets your unique dietary needs and provide ongoing support on your journey.

Arming yourself with the right tools and resources is essential to your macro diet journey. As a beginner, these assets will simplify tracking and inspire you to create balanced, delicious meals that adhere to your macro goals. With these tools at your disposal, you'll find that the world of macros becomes more accessible and enjoyable, allowing you to continue your journey through the Macro Diet with confidence and success.

# Glossary of Macro-Related Terms

Understanding the world of macros is vital to mastering the macro-focused diet.

## 1. Macronutrients (Macros)

Macronutrients are the three main components of your diet that provide energy: carbohydrates, proteins, and fats. Balancing these macros is central to achieving your dietary goals.

## 2. Micronutrients

Micronutrients include vitamins and minerals necessary for various bodily functions, including immune support, energy production, and maintaining healthy skin, hair, and nails.

### 3. Carbohydrates

Carbohydrates are the body's primary source of energy. They come in sugars, starches, and fiber and are found in fruits, vegetables, grains, and legumes.

### 4. Proteins

Proteins are essential for building and repairing tissues, making enzymes, hormones, and other body chemicals. They're found in meat, dairy, legumes, and some grains.

### 5. Fats

Fats are concentrated sources of energy that support brain function and hormone production. Healthy fats can be found in avocados, nuts, seeds, and olive oil.

### 6. Calorie

A calorie is a unit of energy. It measures the power you obtain from a food or beverage when your body breaks it down.

### 7. Calories In vs. Calories Out

This concept involves the balance between the calories you consume and the calories you burn. It's a fundamental principle in weight management.

### 8. Macronutrient Ratio

The ratio of carbohydrates, proteins, and fats in your diet determines your daily macronutrient intake in percentages or grams.

### 9. BMR (Basal Metabolic Rate)

Your BMR is the number of calories your body needs at rest to maintain essential functions like breathing and circulation.

### 10. TDEE (Total Daily Energy Expenditure)

TDEE represents the total calories your body requires daily, accounting for your activity level. It's crucial for calculating your daily caloric intake.

### 11. Fiber

Dietary fiber is a type of carbohydrate found in plant-based foods. It's crucial for digestive health and can help control appetite.

### 12. Net Carbs

Net carbs represent the total carbs in a food item minus the fiber and certain sugar alcohols. They provide a more accurate view of a food's impact on blood sugar.

### 13. Glycemic Index (GI)

The GI measures how quickly a carbohydrate-containing food raises blood sugar levels. Foods with a high GI can cause rapid spikes in blood sugar.

### 14. Insulin

Insulin is a hormone produced by the pancreas that helps regulate blood sugar levels by allowing cells to take in glucose for energy.

### 15. Ketosis

Ketosis is a metabolic state in which the body burns fat for energy instead of carbohydrates. It's commonly associated with low-carb and ketogenic diets.

### 16. Essential Fatty Acids

These are fats that the body cannot produce on its own and must be obtained through the diet. Omega-3 and omega-6 fatty acids are examples of essential fats.

### 17. Lean Protein

Lean proteins are sources of protein with lower fat content. They include skinless poultry, lean cuts of meat, and plant-based proteins like tofu.

## 18. Omega-3 Fatty Acids

Omega-3 fatty acids are polyunsaturated fats known for their heart-healthy benefits. They're found in fatty fish like salmon and in flaxseeds and walnuts.

## 19. Sugar Alcohols

Sugar alcohols are sweeteners found in some sugar-free or low-calorie foods. They have fewer calories than sugar and a reduced impact on blood sugar.

## 20. Meal Prep

Meal prep involves planning and preparing meals in advance. It helps you stick to your dietary goals by having healthy, portion-controlled options readily available.

This glossary serves as a valuable reference as you progress.

# FAQs and Troubleshooting for New Macro Dieters

As you delve into the macro-focused diet, having questions and encountering challenges is common. In this chapter of the Macro Cookbook for Beginners, we'll address frequently asked questions and provide troubleshooting tips to help you navigate your macro journey effectively.

## 1. What Are Macros, and Why Do They Matter?

Macronutrients, or macros, are your body's fundamental nutrients for energy and various bodily functions. They consist of carbohydrates, proteins, and fats. Tracking macros is vital because it allows you to manage your calorie intake, optimize your nutrient balance, and work toward specific dietary and fitness goals.

## 2. How Do I Calculate My Macros?

Calculating macros requires determining your Total Daily Energy Expenditure (TDEE) and then allocating macronutrients based on your goals. Many online calculators can help, or you can consult a registered dietitian for personalized guidance.

## 3. Is It Possible to Eat My Favorite Foods on a Macro Diet?

You can incorporate your favorite foods into a macro diet, provided you do so mindfully. Tracking your macros allows for flexibility, so you can enjoy occasional indulgences while staying within your dietary goals.

## 4. What If I Have Dietary Restrictions or Preferences?

Macro diets are versatile and can accommodate various dietary restrictions or preferences, such as vegan, vegetarian, gluten-free, or low-carb. You can adapt your macros to suit your needs while maintaining balance.

## 5. How Do I Handle Social Situations or Dining Out?

Social events and dining out can be challenging. Still, with some planning and wise choices, you can enjoy these occasions while maintaining your macros. Look for menu options that align with your dietary goals and practice portion control.

## 6. What If I'm Not Seeing Progress?

If you need to see the desired results, it's essential to troubleshoot. Check your calorie and macro tracking for accuracy. Adjust your macros if necessary and ensure you incorporate various nutrient-dense foods into your diet.

## 7. How Can I Overcome Cravings?

Cravings are common. To manage them, opt for healthier versions of your favorite foods or allocate a portion of your daily macros to satisfy your cravings. Drinking water and staying busy can also help curb cravings.

## 8. Can I Adjust My Macros Over Time?

You can and should adjust your macros as your goals or needs change. If you're experiencing a weight loss plateau, for example, consider modifying your macros or calorie intake.

### 9. How Do I Handle Plateaus in My Progress?

Plateaus are natural in any dietary journey. To overcome them, adjust your macros, increase physical activity, or try new recipes to add variety to your diet.

### 10. How Do I Stay Motivated on a Macro Diet?

Staying motivated can be challenging, but setting clear, realistic goals and tracking your progress is essential. Surround yourself with a supportive community or dietitian who can provide guidance and motivation.

Embarking on a macro-focused diet is rewarding, but facing questions and hurdles is common. By addressing these FAQs and providing troubleshooting tips, we aim to equip you with the knowledge and strategies to navigate your dietary journey confidently. Your macro journey is uniquely yours, and with the proper guidance and persistence, you can achieve your nutritional goals and enjoy a healthier, more balanced lifestyle.

# MEAL PLAN

## 2-WEEK MEAL PLAN FOR EFFECTIVE WEIGHT LOSS

Please keep in mind that this is just a sample, and you can adjust portion sizes and ingredients based on your preferences and dietary requirements.

### Week 1:

| DAYS | BREAKFAST | LUNCH | SNACK | DINNER |
|---|---|---|---|---|
| DAY – 1 MONDAY | Avocado and Turkey Breakfast Burrito Page #24 | Creamy Avocado Pesto Pasta Page #34 | Crispy Roasted Chickpeas Page #48 | Lemon Garlic Shrimp Linguine Page #34 |
| DAY – 2 TUESDAY | Sweet Potato and Black Bean Hash with Poached Eggs Page #25 | Mediterranean Orzo Salad Page #38 | Spiced Roasted Edamame Page #50 | Chicken and Broccoli Alfredo Page #35 |
| DAY – 3 WEDNESDAY | Bacon and Veggie Breakfast Skillet Page #26 | Thai-Inspired Peanut Noodle Bowl Page #36 | Almond and Coconut Energy Bites Page #53 | Veggie-Packed Spaghetti Primavera Page #36 |
| DAY – 4 THURSADAY | Mediterranean-Style Quinoa Breakfast Bowl Page #26 | Beef and Mushroom Stroganoff Page #37 | Caprese Skewers with Balsamic Glaze Page #55 | Roasted Red Pepper and Spinach Fettuccine Page #38 |
| DAY – 5 FRIDAY | Vegetable Frittata with a Side of Salsa Page #27 | Pesto Tortellini Salad Page #42 | Turkey and Avocado Roll-Ups Page #50 | Spinach and Ricotta Stuffed Shells Page #41 |
| DAY – 6 SATURDAY | Cheesy Sausage and Zucchini Casserole Page #27 | Creamy Sundried Tomato and Basil Farfalle Page #39 | Smoked Salmon Cucumber Bites Page #53 | Pesto Grilled Shrimp Skewers Page #65 |
| DAY – 7 SUNDAY | Egg White and Spinach Breakfast Quesadilla Page #28 | Spinach and Vegetable Stir-Fry Page #96 | Nut Butter and Banana Sandwich Page #51 | Moroccan-Spiced Rabbit Stew Page #75 |

| DAYS | BREAKFAST | LUNCH | SNACK | DINNER |
|---|---|---|---|---|
| DAY – 8 MONDAY | Quinoa Porridge with Mixed Berries Page #31 | Chicken Piccata with Capers Page #82 | Spicy Buffalo Cauliflower Bites Page #48 | Spinach and Vegetable Stir-Fry Page #96 |
| DAY – 9 TUESDAY | Herbed Tofu Scramble with Tomatoes and Spinach Page #31 | Moroccan Lentil Soup with Spiced Tomato Broth Page #99 | Caprese Skewers with Balsamic Glaze Page #55 | Grilled Swordfish Steaks with Mango Salsa Page #61 |
| DAY – 10 WEDNESDAY | Portobello Mushroom and Egg Breakfast Stack Page #32 | Thai-Inspired Coconut Curry Soup with Tofu Page #100 | Nut Butter and Banana Sandwich Page #51 | Mediterranean-Style Baked Cod Page #62 |
| DAY – 11 THURSADAY | Veggie-Loaded Breakfast Wrap with Lean Turkey Page #33 | Creamy Broccoli and Cheddar Soup Page #99 | Crispy Roasted Chickpeas Page #48 | Thai-Style Coconut Curry Shrimp Page #63 |
| DAY – 12 FRIDAY | Turkey Sausage and Mushroom Breakfast Strata Page #30 | Spiced Carrot and Ginger Soup Page #102 | Almond and Coconut Energy Bites Page #53 | Teriyaki Glazed Salmon with Sesame Broccoli Page #63 |
| DAY – 13 SATURDAY | Quinoa and Black Bean Stuffed Peppers Page #51 | Vegan Split Pea Soup with Smoked Paprika Page #103 | Turkey and Avocado Roll-Ups Page #50 | Herb-Crusted Baked Halibut Page #64 |
| DAY – 14 SUNDAY | Chimichurri Marinated Grilled Tuna Page #66 | Roasted Red Pepper and Chickpea Soup Page #104 | Caprese Skewers with Balsamic Glaze Page #55 | Pesto Grilled Shrimp Skewers Page #65 |

This meal plan incorporates a variety of foods to help you stay on track with your weight loss goals. Make sure to control portion sizes, drink plenty of water, and incorporate regular physical activity into your routine for the best results.

Remember that individual calorie needs can vary, so it's a good idea to consult with a registered dietitian or nutritionist to customize a meal plan that aligns with your specific goals and preferences.

# Tips for Effective Weight Loss:

1.  **Mindful Eating:** Pay attention to your body's hunger and fullness cues. Eat slowly, savoring each bite, and stop when you feel satisfied, not stuffed.

2.  **Balanced Meals:** Aim for balanced meals that include lean proteins, whole grains, healthy fats, and plenty of vegetables. This balance provides essential nutrients while keeping you full longer.

3.  **Portion Control:** Use smaller plates and bowls to help control portion sizes. This can prevent overeating and encourage mindful consumption.

4.  **Stay Hydrated:** Drink water throughout the day. Sometimes, feelings of hunger are actually signs of dehydration. Keeping hydrated supports your metabolism and overall well-being.

5.  **Limit Processed Foods:** Minimize your intake of processed foods, sugary snacks, and sweetened beverages. These often contain hidden calories and lack essential nutrients.

6.  **Regular Exercise:** Incorporate regular physical activity into your routine. Find activities you enjoy, whether it's walking, dancing, or cycling. Exercise not only burns calories but also boosts your mood and energy levels.

7.  **Healthy Snacking:** Opt for nutritious snacks like fresh fruits, vegetables with hummus, or a handful of nuts. Healthy snacks can prevent overeating during main meals.

8.  **Sleep Well:** Aim for 7-9 hours of sleep each night. Lack of sleep can disrupt hormones related to hunger and stress, leading to weight gain.

9.  **Manage Stress:** Practice stress-reducing activities such as yoga, meditation, or deep breathing exercises. Stress can lead to emotional eating and cravings for unhealthy foods.

10. **Track Progress:** Keep a food journal or use a mobile app to track your meals, exercise, and emotions related to eating. Monitoring your progress can help you identify patterns and make necessary adjustments.

11. **Support System:** Surround yourself with supportive friends and family who encourage your healthy habits. Consider joining a fitness class or online community for added motivation.

12. **Celebrate Achievements:** Celebrate your successes, no matter how small. Rewarding yourself positively reinforces your efforts and keeps you motivated.

13. **Consult a Professional:** If you find it challenging to lose weight, consider consulting a registered dietitian or a healthcare provider. They can provide personalized guidance and support tailored to your needs.

Remember, every person's body is different, so what works for one may not work for another. It's crucial to find a balance that fits your lifestyle and preferences. Stay patient, stay consistent, and focus on building sustainable, healthy habits for long-term success.

# 2-WEEK MUSCLE MASS RECRUITMENT MEAL PLAN

## Week 1:

| DAYS | BREAKFAST | LUNCH | SNACK | DINNER |
|---|---|---|---|---|
| **DAY – 1**<br>**MONDAY** | Avocado and Turkey Breakfast Burrito<br>Page #24 | Lemon Garlic Shrimp Linguine<br>Page #34 | Almond and Coconut Energy Bites<br>Page #53 | Grilled Turkey Burgers with Avocado<br>Page #73 |
| **DAY – 2**<br>**TUESDAY** | Cheesy Sausage and Zucchini Casserole<br>Page #27 | Chicken and Broccoli Alfredo<br>Page #35 | Smoked Salmon Cucumber Bites<br>Page #53 | Mediterranean-Style Baked Cod<br>Page #62 |
| **DAY – 3**<br>**WEDNESDAY** | Spinach and Feta Stuffed Omelette<br>Page #24 | Veggie-Packed Spaghetti Primavera<br>Page #36 | Nut Butter and Banana Sandwich<br>Page #51 | Thai-Inspired Coconut Curry Shrimp<br>Page #63 |
| **DAY – 4**<br>**THURSADAY** | Protein-Packed Cottage Cheese Pancakes<br>Page #29 | Beef and Mushroom Stroganoff<br>Page #37 | Crispy Roasted Chickpeas<br>Page #48 | Herb-Crusted Baked Halibut<br>Page #64 |
| **DAY – 5**<br>**FRIDAY** | Breakfast Stuffed Bell Peppers<br>Page #29 | Roasted Red Pepper and Spinach Fettuccine<br>Page #38 | Caprese Skewers with Balsamic Glaze<br>Page #55 | Teriyaki Glazed Salmon with Sesame Broccoli<br>Page #63 |
| **DAY – 6**<br>**SATURDAY** | Quinoa Porridge with Mixed Berries<br>Page #31 | Pesto Tortellini Salad<br>Page #42 | Spiced Roasted Edamame<br>Page #50 | Mediterranean Zucchini and Shrimp Stir-Fry<br>Page #68 |
| **DAY – 7**<br>**SUNDAY** | Portobello Mushroom and Egg Breakfast Stack<br>Page #32 | Creamy Sundried Tomato and Basil Farfalle<br>Page #39 | Avocado and Black Bean Salsa<br>Page #49 | Lemon-Dill Baked Trout with Steamed Greens<br>Page #67 |

Week 2:

| DAYS | BREAKFAST | LUNCH | SNACK | DINNER |
|---|---|---|---|---|
| DAY – 8 MONDAY | Vegetable Frittata with a Side of Salsa Page #27 | Turkey and Spinach Lasagna Page #40 | Cottage Cheese with Pineapple and Walnuts Page #52 | Miso-Glazed Cod with Roasted Brussels Sprouts Page #67 |
| DAY – 9 TUESDAY | Egg White and Spinach Breakfast Quesadilla Page #28 | Spicy Cajun Shrimp Pasta Page #41 | BBQ Pulled Chicken Sliders Page #56 | Mediterranean-Style Veal Scaloppini Page #84 |
| DAY – 10 WEDNESDAY | Herbed Tofu Scramble with Tomatoes and Spinach Page #31 | Spinach and Ricotta Stuffed Shells Page #41 | Caprese Baguette with Pesto Mayo Page #58 | Quail and Wild Mushroom Risotto Page #85 |
| DAY – 11 THURSADAY | Veggie-Loaded Breakfast Wrap with Lean Turkey Page #33 | Pesto Grilled Shrimp Skewers Page #65 | Crispy Roasted Chickpeas Page #48 | Grilled Quail with Rosemary and Garlic Page #85 |
| DAY – 12 FRIDAY | Turkey Sausage and Mushroom Breakfast Strata Page #30 | Spinach and Vegetable Stir-Fry Page #96 | Turkey and Avocado Roll-Ups Page #50 | Braised Veal Osso Buco Page #86 |
| DAY – 13 SATURDAY | Mediterranean-Style Quinoa Breakfast Bowl Page #26 | Thai-Style Coconut Curry Shrimp Page #63 | Quinoa and Black Bean Stuffed Peppers Page #51 | Chimichurri Marinated Grilled Tuna Page #66 |
| DAY – 14 SUNDAY | Veggie-Loaded Breakfast Wrap with Lean Turkey Page #33 | Tuna and White Bean Salad Page #45 | Caprese Skewers with Balsamic Glaze Page #55 | Lemon-Rosemary Roasted Chicken Page #73 |

Ensure to adjust portion sizes based on your activity level and consult with a nutritionist or fitness expert for personalized adjustments to meet your specific muscle recruitment goals. Stay hydrated and engage in regular physical activity to optimize your results.

# Tips for Effective Muscle Mass Recruitment:

1.  **Stay Hydrated:** Drink plenty of water throughout the day to support muscle function and recovery. Dehydration can hinder your progress.

2.  **Balanced Nutrition:** Ensure a balance of macronutrients in your meals—protein, carbohydrates, and healthy fats are crucial for muscle development.

3.  **Consistent Protein Intake:** Incorporate lean protein sources in every meal to provide your muscles with the amino acids they need to grow and recover.

4.  **Regular Exercise:** Combine your meal plan with a well-structured exercise routine that includes both resistance and cardiovascular training.

5.  **Monitor Progress:** Keep a journal to track your meals, exercises, and physical progress. Adjust your plan as needed based on your results.

6.  **Get Plenty of Rest:** Allow your muscles to recover with adequate sleep and rest days between intense workouts.

7.  **Consult a Professional:** If you have specific muscle recruitment goals, consider working with a fitness expert or dietitian for a personalized plan and guidance.

Remember that building muscle is a gradual process. Be patient and consistent with your nutrition and exercise to achieve your desired results.

# BREAKFAST

## Avocado and Turkey Breakfast Burrito

Serving: 4 | Prep time: 15 minutes | Cook time: 10 minutes

Ingredients:

- 8 oz (225 g) lean ground turkey
- 1 tsp olive oil
- 4 large eggs
- 1 ripe avocado, diced
- 4 whole wheat tortillas (8-inch/20 cm)
- 4 oz (115 g) reduced-fat cheddar cheese, shredded
- 4 tbsp salsa
- Salt and pepper to taste

Directions:

1. In a skillet, heat the olive oil over medium heat. Add the ground turkey, and cook until browned and cooked through, breaking it into small pieces as it cooks, for about 5-7 minutes. Season with a pinch of salt and pepper.
2. In a separate pan, scramble the eggs over medium heat until just set. Remove from heat and set aside.
3. Warm the tortillas in the microwave for 20 seconds or in a dry skillet until pliable.
4. Assemble the burritos: Lay out each tortilla, and evenly distribute the cooked turkey, scrambled eggs, diced avocado, shredded cheddar cheese, and salsa in the center of each tortilla.
5. Fold the sides of the tortilla over the filling, then fold the bottom up and roll tightly to create the burrito.
6. Return the burrito to the skillet over medium heat and cook for 2-3 minutes on each side until it's lightly toasted and the cheese is melted.

Nutritional Values: Calories: 320 kcal | Fat: 17 g | Protein: 22 g | Carbs: 22 g | Net carbs: 15 g | Fiber: 7 g | Cholesterol: 195 mg | Sodium: 460 mg | Potassium: 670 mg

Useful Tip: Customize your breakfast burrito with additional ingredients like diced tomatoes, black beans, or a sprinkle of cilantro for added flavor and nutrition. Enjoy the dish!

## Spinach and Feta Stuffed Omelette

Serving: 4 | Prep time: 10 minutes | Cook time: 10 minutes

Ingredients:

- 8 large eggs
- 4 oz (115 g) fresh baby spinach, chopped
- 2 oz (57 g) crumbled feta cheese
- 2 oz (60 ml) skim milk
- 2 tsp olive oil
- Salt and pepper to taste

Directions:

1. In a bowl, whisk together the eggs, skim milk, and a pinch of salt and pepper.
2. Heat 1/2 teaspoon of olive oil in a non-stick skillet over medium heat. Add a quarter of the chopped spinach and sauté until wilted.

3. Pour a quarter of the egg mixture into the skillet, swirling it around to create an even layer. Cook until the edges start to set.
4. Sprinkle a quarter of the crumbled feta cheese over one-half of the omelette.
5. Carefully fold the other half of the omelette over the cheese. Cook for an additional 1-2 minutes until the cheese melts, and the omelette is cooked through.
6. Slide the omelette onto a plate, and repeat the process for the remaining three omelettes.

**Nutritional Values:** Calories: 220 kcal | Fat: 15 g | Protein: 14 g | Carbs: 5 g | Net carbs: 4 g | Fiber: 1 g | Cholesterol: 380 mg | Sodium: 430 mg | Potassium: 300 mg

**Useful Tip:** You can customize your omelette by adding diced tomatoes, sautéed mushrooms, or bell peppers for extra flavor and nutrients. Enjoy the dish!

## Sweet Potato and Black Bean Hash with Poached Eggs

Serving: 4 | Prep time: 15 minutes | Cook time: 20 minutes

**Ingredients:**

- 16 oz (450 g) sweet potatoes, peeled and diced
- 1 can (15 oz / 425 g) black beans, drained and rinsed
- 4 large eggs
- 2 tbsp olive oil
- 1 small onion, diced
- 1 red bell pepper, diced
- 1 tsp ground cumin
- 1/2 tsp chili powder
- Salt and pepper to taste

**Directions:**

1. In a large skillet, heat the olive oil over medium-high heat. Add the diced sweet potatoes and sauté for about 10 minutes, or until they are tender and slightly crispy.
2. Add the diced onion and red bell pepper to the skillet, and cook for an additional 3-4 minutes until they are softened and slightly caramelized.
3. Stir in the ground cumin and chili powder, and add the black beans. Cook for another 2-3 minutes until everything is well combined and heated through. Season with salt and pepper to taste.
4. Meanwhile, poach the eggs. Bring a pot of water to a gentle simmer, and add a splash of vinegar. Crack each egg into a small cup or ramekin and carefully slide them into the simmering water. Cook for about 3-4 minutes for runny yolks or longer for firmer yolks.
5. Divide the sweet potato and black bean hash among four plates, and place a poached egg on top of each serving.

**Nutritional Values:** Calories: 280 kcal | Fat: 9 g | Protein: 11 g | Carbs: 40 g | Net carbs: 11 g | Fiber: 9 g | Cholesterol: 185 mg | Sodium: 450 mg | Potassium: 650 mg

**Useful Tip:** Customize your hash by adding diced avocado, salsa, or a dollop of Greek yogurt for extra flavor and creaminess. Enjoy the dish!

# Bacon and Veggie Breakfast Skillet

Serving: 4 | Prep time: 10 minutes | Cook time: 20 minutes

Ingredients:

- 8 oz (225 g) bacon, chopped
- 4 large eggs
- 1 bell pepper, diced
- 1 small onion, diced
- 1 zucchini, diced
- 4 oz (115 g) cherry tomatoes, halved
- 2 oz (60 ml) milk
- Salt and pepper to taste

Directions:

1. In a large skillet, cook the chopped bacon over medium heat until it becomes crispy and golden brown. Remove it from the skillet and place it on paper towels to drain excess grease.
2. In the same skillet, without cleaning it, add the diced onion and bell pepper. Sauté for about 3-4 minutes until they start to soften.
3. Stir in the diced zucchini and cherry tomatoes, and continue cooking for an additional 3-4 minutes until the vegetables are tender.
4. In a bowl, whisk the eggs and milk together, then pour the mixture into the skillet with the vegetables. Stir gently to combine, and cook until the eggs are set but still slightly runny.
5. Sprinkle the crispy bacon over the top, season with salt and pepper to taste, and cook for another 1-2 minutes to warm the bacon.

**Nutritional Values:** Calories: 290 kcal | Fat: 18 g | Protein: 16 g | Carbs: 12 g | Net carbs: 8 g | Fiber: 4 g | Cholesterol: 250 mg | Sodium: 650 mg | Potassium: 700 mg

**Useful Tip:** For a spicy kick, add a pinch of red pepper flakes or a dash of hot sauce to the skillet when sautéing the veggies. Enjoy the dish!

# Mediterranean-Style Quinoa Breakfast Bowl

Serving: 4 | Prep time: 15 minutes | Cook time: 20 minutes

Ingredients:

- 8 oz (225 g) quinoa
- 16 oz (475 ml) water
- 16 oz (450 g) cherry tomatoes, halved
- 4 large eggs
- 4 oz (115 g) cucumber, diced
- 4 oz (115 g) feta cheese, crumbled
- 2 oz (60 ml) extra virgin olive oil
- 2 oz (60 ml) fresh lemon juice
- 2 tsp dried oregano
- Salt and pepper to taste

Directions:

1. Rinse the quinoa under cold water. In a saucepan, combine the quinoa with 2 cups (475 ml) of water. Bring to a boil, then reduce the heat, cover, and simmer for about 15 minutes or until the quinoa is cooked and the water is absorbed. Remove from heat and let it cool.
2. In a small bowl, whisk together the olive oil, lemon juice, dried oregano, salt, and pepper to create the dressing.

3. In a large mixing bowl, combine the cooked quinoa, halved cherry tomatoes, diced cucumber, and crumbled feta cheese. Toss the ingredients together.

4. In a separate skillet, cook the eggs to your liking (poached or fried).

5. Divide the quinoa mixture among four bowls, top each with a cooked egg, and drizzle the dressing over the top.

**Nutritional Values:** Calories: 380 kcal | Fat: 22 g | Protein: 14 g | Carbs: 30 g | Net carbs: 24 g | Fiber: 6 g | Cholesterol: 195 mg | Sodium: 420 mg | Potassium: 500 mg

**Useful Tip:** Add some chopped kalamata olives and a sprinkle of fresh parsley for an extra burst of Mediterranean flavor. Enjoy the dish!

## Vegetable Frittata with a Side of Salsa

Serving: 4 | Prep time: 15 minutes | Cook time: 25 minutes

**Ingredients:**

- 8 large eggs
- 4 oz (115 g) bell peppers, diced
- 4 oz (115 g) zucchini, diced
- 4 oz (115 g) cherry tomatoes, halved
- 2 oz (60 ml) milk
- 2 oz (60 ml) salsa
- 2 oz (60 g) shredded cheddar cheese
- 2 tsp olive oil
- Salt and pepper to taste

**Directions:**

1. Preheat your oven to 350°F (175°C).

2. In an oven-safe skillet, heat the olive oil over medium heat. Add the diced bell peppers and zucchini, and sauté for about 5 minutes until they start to soften.

3. In a bowl, whisk together the eggs, milk, salt, and pepper. Pour this mixture into the skillet with the sautéed vegetables.

4. Add the halved cherry tomatoes and shredded cheddar cheese to the skillet, distributing them evenly.

5. Transfer the skillet to the preheated oven and bake for approximately 20 minutes or until the frittata is set and the top is lightly browned.

6. Serve it with a side of salsa for an extra burst of flavor.

**Nutritional Values:** Calories: 280 kcal | Fat: 19 g | Protein: 16 g | Carbs: 11 g | Net carbs: 8 g | Fiber: 3 g | Cholesterol: 370 mg | Sodium: 420 mg | Potassium: 450 mg

**Useful Tip:** You can customize your frittata with your favorite vegetables and herbs like spinach, onions, or basil. Enjoy the dish!

## Cheesy Sausage and Zucchini Casserole

Serving: 4 | Prep time: 20 minutes | Cook time: 35 minutes

**Ingredients:**

- 12 oz (340 g) ground sausage
- 8 oz (225 g) zucchini, diced
- 4 oz (115 g) cheddar cheese, shredded
- 4 large eggs

- 2 oz (60 ml) heavy cream
- 2 oz (60 ml) unsweetened almond milk
- 1/2 tsp garlic powder
- Salt and pepper to taste

Directions:

1. Preheat your oven to 375°F (190°C).
2. In a skillet, cook the ground sausage over medium-high heat until browned and cooked through, breaking it into crumbles as it cooks.
3. In a bowl, whisk together the eggs, heavy cream, almond milk, garlic powder, salt, and pepper.
4. Grease a baking dish and spread the cooked sausage and diced zucchini evenly in the dish.
5. Pour the egg mixture over the sausage and zucchini, then sprinkle the shredded cheddar cheese on top.
6. Bake in the preheated oven for about 30-35 minutes or until the casserole is set in the center and the cheese is melted and bubbly.

Nutritional Values: Calories: 380 kcal | Fat: 30 g | Protein: 20 g | Carbs: 4 g | Net carbs: 3 g | Fiber: 1 g | Cholesterol: 230 mg | Sodium: 560 mg | Potassium: 280 mg

Useful Tip: Customize your casserole by adding your favorite herbs and spices, like fresh basil or paprika, to enhance the flavors. Enjoy the dish!

## Egg White and Spinach Breakfast Quesadilla

Serving: 4 | Prep time: 10 minutes | Cook time: 15 minutes

Ingredients:

- 8 large egg whites
- 4 whole wheat tortillas (8-inch/20 cm)
- 4 oz (115 g) baby spinach
- 4 oz (115 g) reduced-fat mozzarella cheese, shredded
- 2 oz (60 ml) salsa
- 2 tsp olive oil
- Salt and pepper to taste

Directions:

1. In a non-stick skillet, heat 1/2 teaspoon of olive oil over medium heat. Add the baby spinach and sauté until wilted. Remove from the skillet and set aside.
2. Wipe the skillet clean and heat the remaining 1.5 teaspoons of olive oil over medium heat. Pour in the egg whites, salt, pepper and cook, stirring occasionally until they are set but still slightly runny.
3. Lay out each tortilla and evenly distribute the cooked egg whites, sautéed spinach, shredded mozzarella cheese, and salsa on one half of each tortilla.
4. Fold the other half of the tortilla over the filling to create a half-moon shape.
5. Return the quesadilla to the skillet over medium heat and cook for 2-3 minutes on each side until it's lightly toasted and the cheese is melted.

Nutritional Values: Calories: 240 kcal | Fat: 8 g | Protein: 22 g | Carbs: 20 g | Net carbs: 14 g | Fiber: 6 g | Cholesterol: 10 mg | Sodium: 490 mg | Potassium: 380 mg

Useful Tip: Customize your quesadilla with diced tomatoes, black beans, or a sprinkle of cilantro for added flavor and nutrition. Enjoy the dish!

# Protein-Packed Cottage Cheese Pancakes

Serving: 4 | Prep time: 10 minutes | Cook time: 15 minutes

Ingredients:

- 16 oz (450 g) low-fat cottage cheese
- 4 large eggs
- 4 oz (115 g) oat flour
- 2 oz (60 ml) almond milk
- 1 tsp vanilla extract
- 2 tsp honey (optional)
- 1/2 tsp baking powder
- 1/4 tsp salt
- Cooking spray

Directions:

1. In a blender, combine the low-fat cottage cheese, eggs, oat flour, almond milk, vanilla extract, honey (if using), baking powder, and salt. Blend until you have a smooth, pancake batter.
2. Preheat a non-stick skillet over medium heat and lightly grease it with cooking spray.
3. Pour 1/4 cup of the pancake batter onto the skillet for each pancake. Cook for 2-3 minutes on one side until you see bubbles on the surface, then flip and cook for another 1-2 minutes until they're golden brown.
4. Remove the pancakes from the skillet and keep them warm. Repeat with the remaining batter.

**Nutritional Values:** Calories: 280 kcal | Fat: 6 g | Protein: 26 g | Carbs: 30 g | Net carbs: 24 g | Fiber: 6 g | Cholesterol: 190 mg | Sodium: 650 mg | Potassium: 370 mg

**Useful Tip:** These pancakes are versatile. Top them with fresh berries, Greek yogurt, or a drizzle of pure maple syrup for added flavor. Enjoy the dish!

# Breakfast Stuffed Bell Peppers

Serving: 4 | Prep time: 15 minutes | Cook time: 40 minutes

Ingredients:

- 4 bell peppers
- 8 large eggs
- 4 oz (115 g) ground breakfast sausage
- 4 oz (115 g) cherry tomatoes, diced
- 4 oz (115 g) spinach, chopped
- 2 oz (60 ml) milk
- 4 oz (120 ml) shredded cheddar cheese
- Salt and pepper to taste

Directions:

1. Preheat your oven to 375°F (190°C).
2. Cut the tops off the bell peppers, remove the seeds and membranes, and set them aside.
3. In a skillet over medium heat, cook the breakfast sausage until it's browned and cooked through. Remove excess grease, leaving a little for flavor.
4. Add the diced cherry tomatoes and chopped spinach to the skillet with the sausage. Sauté for a few minutes until the spinach wilts and the tomatoes soften.
5. In a bowl, whisk together the eggs, milk, salt, and pepper. Pour the egg mixture into the skillet with the sausage and vegetables. Cook, stirring occasionally, until the eggs are set but still slightly runny.
6. Stuff each bell pepper with the egg and sausage mixture, and top each with shredded cheddar cheese.

7.  Place the stuffed bell peppers in a baking dish and bake in the preheated oven for 20-25 minutes or until the peppers are tender and the cheese is bubbly and golden.

**Nutritional Values:** Calories: 270 kcal | Fat: 16 g | Protein: 21 g | Carbs: 13 g | Net carbs: 8 g | Fiber: 5 g | Cholesterol: 360 mg | Sodium: 450 mg | Potassium: 670 mg

**Useful Tip:** You can add your favorite spices and herbs to the egg mixture for extra flavor. Enjoy the dish!

## Turkey Sausage and Mushroom Breakfast Strata

Serving: 4 | Prep time: 20 minutes | Cook time: 45 minutes

**Ingredients:**

- 8 oz (225 g) whole wheat bread, cubed
- 4 oz (115 g) lean turkey sausage, crumbled
- 4 oz (115 g) mushrooms, sliced
- 2 oz (60 g) shredded low-fat cheddar cheese
- 6 large eggs
- 2 oz (60 ml) unsweetened almond milk
- 2 oz (60 ml) low-sodium vegetable broth
- 1 tsp olive oil
- 1/2 tsp dried thyme
- Salt and pepper to taste

**Directions:**

1.  Preheat your oven to 350°F (175°C).
2.  In a skillet, heat the olive oil over medium heat. Add the crumbled turkey sausage and cook until browned. Remove the cooked sausage and set it aside.
3.  In the same skillet, add the sliced mushrooms and sauté until they release their moisture and become tender, about 5 minutes. Remove from heat.
4.  In a bowl, whisk together the eggs, almond milk, low-sodium vegetable broth, dried thyme, salt, and pepper.
5.  In a greased baking dish, place the cubed whole wheat bread, cooked turkey sausage, sautéed mushrooms, and shredded low-fat cheddar cheese.
6.  Pour the egg mixture over the bread and other ingredients, ensuring everything is evenly coated.
7.  Bake in the preheated oven for about 40-45 minutes or until the strata is set in the center and the top is golden and slightly crispy.

**Nutritional Values:** Calories: 290 kcal | Fat: 10 g | Protein: 21 g | Carbs: 25 g | Net carbs: 20 g | Fiber: 5 g | Cholesterol: 280 mg | Sodium: 560 mg | Potassium: 370 mg

**Useful Tip:** You can prepare this strata the night before and refrigerate it, then bake it in the morning for a quick and delicious breakfast. Enjoy the dish!

# Quinoa Porridge with Mixed Berries

Serving: 4 | Prep time: 10 minutes | Cook time: 20 minutes

Ingredients:

- 8 oz (225 g) quinoa
- 2 oz (60 g) mixed berries (blueberries, strawberries, raspberries)
- 2 oz (60 g) almonds, chopped
- 4 oz (115 g) Greek yogurt
- 2 oz (60 ml) honey
- 1/2 tsp ground cinnamon
- 2 oz (60 ml) unsweetened almond milk
- 2 oz (60 ml) water
- 2 oz (60 ml) orange juice
- 1/2 tsp vanilla extract
- A pinch of salt

Directions:

1. Rinse the quinoa under cold water until the water runs clear.
2. In a saucepan, combine the rinsed quinoa, water, and a pinch of salt. Bring to a boil, then reduce the heat to low, cover, and simmer for 15-20 minutes, or until the quinoa is tender and the liquid is absorbed. Remove from heat.
3. While the quinoa is still warm, stir in the unsweetened almond milk, orange juice, honey, and vanilla extract.
4. Divide the quinoa mixture into serving bowls and top with mixed berries, chopped almonds, and a dollop of Greek yogurt.
5. Sprinkle ground cinnamon over each bowl for added flavor.

**Nutritional Values:** Calories: 290 kcal | Fat: 8 g | Protein: 10 g | Carbs: 45 g | Net carbs: 35 g | Fiber: 5 g | Cholesterol: 2 mg | Sodium: 60 mg | Potassium: 330 mg

**Useful Tip:** Customize your quinoa porridge by adding your favorite nuts, seeds, or sweeteners like maple syrup. Enjoy the dish!

# Herbed Tofu Scramble with Tomatoes and Spinach

Serving: 4 | Prep time: 10 minutes | Cook time: 15 minutes

Ingredients:

- 16 oz (450 g) extra-firm tofu, crumbled
- 4 oz (115 g) cherry tomatoes, halved
- 4 oz (115 g) fresh spinach
- 2 oz (60 ml) unsweetened almond milk
- 2 oz (60 g) onion, chopped
- 1 oz (30 ml) olive oil
- 1/2 tsp ground turmeric
- 1/2 tsp dried thyme
- Salt and pepper to taste
- A pinch of red pepper flakes

Directions:

1. In a skillet, heat the olive oil over medium heat. Add the chopped onion and sauté until it becomes translucent.
2. Add the crumbled tofu and sprinkle it with ground turmeric, dried thyme, salt, and pepper. Sauté for 3-5 minutes, stirring occasionally until the tofu begins to brown.
3. Stir in the halved cherry tomatoes and cook for another 2 minutes.
4. Add the fresh spinach and continue to cook, stirring frequently until the spinach wilts and the tomatoes soften.

5. Pour in the unsweetened almond milk and a pinch of red pepper flakes for a touch of heat. Cook for an additional 2 minutes until the mixture thickens slightly.

**Nutritional Values:** Calories: 190 kcal | Fat: 12 g | Protein: 15 g | Carbs: 9 g | Net carbs: 4 g | Fiber: 5 g | Cholesterol: 0 mg | Sodium: 180 mg | Potassium: 540 mg

**Useful Tip:** Customize your tofu scramble with your favorite herbs and spices, such as nutritional yeast for a cheesy flavor or smoked paprika for a smoky twist. Enjoy the dish!

# Portobello Mushroom and Egg Breakfast Stack

Serving: 4 | Prep time: 15 minutes | Cook time: 20 minutes

**Ingredients:**

- 4 large Portobello mushrooms
- 4 large eggs
- 4 oz (115 g) spinach
- 2 oz (60 g) red bell pepper, finely chopped
- 2 oz (60 g) feta cheese, crumbled
- 2 oz (60 ml) olive oil
- 1 tsp dried oregano
- Salt and pepper to taste
- Fresh basil leaves for garnish

**Directions:**

1. Preheat your oven to 375°F (190°C).
2. Clean the Portobello mushrooms and remove the stems. Brush the caps with olive oil, sprinkle with dried oregano, and season with salt and pepper.
3. Place the seasoned mushrooms on a baking sheet and bake for 10-12 minutes until they start to soften.
4. While the mushrooms are in the oven, heat the remaining olive oil in a skillet over medium heat. Add the finely chopped red bell pepper and sauté for a few minutes until it softens.
5. Add the spinach to the skillet and cook until it wilts. Season with salt and pepper.
6. Remove the mushrooms from the oven and carefully crack an egg into each cap. Place the baking sheet back in the oven and bake for another 8-10 minutes until the egg whites are set.
7. While the eggs are baking, divide the sautéed spinach and red bell pepper mixture among four plates.
8. Carefully transfer the Portobello mushrooms with baked eggs onto each plate on top of the spinach and red bell pepper mixture.
9. Sprinkle crumbled feta cheese over each stack and garnish with fresh basil leaves.

**Nutritional Values:** Calories: 210 kcal | Fat: 15 g | Protein: 11 g | Carbs: 9 g | Net carbs: 5 g | Fiber: 4 g | Cholesterol: 190 mg | Sodium: 290 mg | Potassium: 640 mg

**Useful Tip:** You can add diced tomatoes, avocado, or a drizzle of balsamic glaze for extra flavor and customization. Enjoy the dish!

# Veggie-Loaded Breakfast Wrap with Lean Turkey

Serving: 4 | Prep time: 15 minutes | Cook time: 10 minutes

## Ingredients:

- 8 oz (225 g) lean ground turkey
- 4 large whole-grain tortillas
- 4 large eggs
- 4 oz (115 g) bell peppers, diced
- 4 oz (115 g) onions, finely chopped
- 2 oz (60 g) spinach leaves
- 2 oz (60 g) low-fat shredded cheddar cheese
- 2 oz (60 ml) salsa
- 2 oz (60 ml) low-fat Greek yogurt
- 2 oz (60 ml) olive oil
- 1/2 tsp chili powder
- Salt and pepper to taste

## Directions:

1. In a skillet, heat olive oil over medium heat. Add the chopped onions and diced bell peppers. Sauté until they become tender, about 4-5 minutes.
2. Add the lean ground turkey to the skillet, breaking it up with a spoon and cooking until browned. Sprinkle with chili powder, salt, and pepper.
3. Push the turkey and vegetable mixture to one side of the skillet, and crack the eggs into the other side. Scramble the eggs with a spatula until they're cooked through.
4. Lay out the whole-grain tortillas and distribute the cooked turkey mixture, scrambled eggs, and a handful of spinach on each tortilla.
5. Sprinkle low-fat shredded cheddar cheese over the fillings on each tortilla.
6. Drizzle salsa and low-fat Greek yogurt over the fillings.
7. Fold in the sides of each tortilla and then roll them up from the bottom, creating a wrap.

**Nutritional Values:** Calories: 320 kcal | Fat: 14 g | Protein: 26 g | Carbs: 22 g | Net carbs: 18 g | Fiber: 4 g | Cholesterol: 180 mg | Sodium: 420 mg | Potassium: 540 mg

**Useful Tip:** These wraps can be customized with your choice of vegetables, and you can adjust the spice level by adding hot sauce or jalapeños. Enjoy the dish!

# PASTA & SALADS

## Creamy Avocado Pesto Pasta

Serving: 4 | Prep time: 15 minutes | Cook time: 12 minutes

Ingredients:

- 12 oz (340 g) whole wheat pasta
- 2 ripe avocados, peeled and pitted
- 2 oz (60 g) fresh basil leaves
- 2 oz (60 g) baby spinach
- 2 oz (60 g) pine nuts
- 2 oz (60 ml) olive oil
- 2 oz (60 ml) lemon juice
- 2 oz (60 g) grated Parmesan cheese
- 2 cloves garlic, minced
- Salt and pepper to taste

Directions:

1. Cook the whole wheat pasta according to package instructions until al dente. Drain and set aside.
2. In a food processor, combine the ripe avocados, fresh basil leaves, baby spinach, pine nuts, olive oil, lemon juice, grated Parmesan cheese, minced garlic, salt, and pepper. Blend until the mixture becomes a smooth, creamy pesto.
3. In a large mixing bowl, toss the cooked pasta with the creamy avocado pesto until the pasta is well coated.
4. Serve the avocado pesto pasta in individual dishes, garnishing with extra grated Parmesan cheese, if desired.

Nutritional Values: Calories: 450 kcal | Fat: 25 g | Protein: 12 g | Carbs: 48 g | Net carbs: 38 g | Fiber: 10 g | Cholesterol: 5 mg | Sodium: 150 mg | Potassium: 620 mg

Useful Tip: You can add grilled chicken, shrimp, or roasted cherry tomatoes for additional protein and flavor. Enjoy the dish!

## Lemon Garlic Shrimp Linguine

Serving: 4 | Prep time: 10 minutes | Cook time: 15 minutes

Ingredients:

- 12 oz (340 g) linguine pasta
- 16 oz (450 g) large shrimp, peeled and deveined
- 2 oz (60 ml) olive oil
- 4 cloves garlic, minced
- Zest of 1 lemon
- Juice of 1 lemon
- 2 oz (60 ml) white wine (optional)
- 2 oz (60 ml) chicken or vegetable broth
- 2 oz (60 g) grated Parmesan cheese
- 2 oz (60 g) fresh parsley, chopped
- Salt and pepper to taste
- Red pepper flakes (optional, for added heat)

Directions:

1. Cook the linguine pasta according to package instructions until al dente. Drain and set aside.
2. In a large skillet, heat olive oil over medium heat. Add the minced garlic and sauté for about 1 minute until fragrant.

3. Add the shrimp to the skillet and cook for 2-3 minutes on each side until they turn pink and opaque. Remove the shrimp from the skillet and set them aside.
4. In the same skillet, add the white wine (if using) and cook for 2 minutes, allowing it to reduce slightly.
5. Stir in the chicken or vegetable broth, lemon zest, and lemon juice. Cook for an additional 2 minutes to combine the flavors.
6. Return the cooked shrimp to the skillet and add the drained linguine pasta. Toss everything together to coat the pasta with the sauce.
7. Stir in grated Parmesan cheese and fresh chopped parsley. Season with salt, pepper, and red pepper flakes (if desired).

**Nutritional Values:** Calories: 450 kcal | Fat: 15 g | Protein: 30 g | Carbs: 40 g | Net carbs: 35 g | Fiber: 5 g | Cholesterol: 180 mg | Sodium: 350 mg | Potassium: 380 mg

**Useful Tip:** For a healthier option, you can use whole wheat linguine pasta. Enjoy the dish!

# Chicken and Broccoli Alfredo

Serving: 4 | Prep time: 15 minutes | Cook time: 20 minutes

## Ingredients:

- 12 oz (340 g) fettuccine pasta
- 16 oz (450 g) boneless, skinless chicken breasts, cut into bite-sized pieces
- 8 oz (225 g) broccoli florets
- 2 oz (60 g) unsalted butter
- 2 oz (60 g) all-purpose flour
- 16 oz (480 ml) whole milk
- 4 oz (120 g) grated Parmesan cheese
- 2 oz (60 g) grated mozzarella cheese
- 2 cloves garlic, minced
- Salt and pepper to taste
- 2 oz (60 ml) chicken broth
- 2 oz (60 ml) white wine (optional)
- Fresh parsley, for garnish

## Directions:

1. Cook the fettuccine pasta according to package instructions until al dente. Add the broccoli florets to the boiling pasta water in the last 3 minutes of cooking. Drain and set aside.
2. In a large skillet, heat the unsalted butter over medium heat. Add the chicken pieces and cook until they are no longer pink, about 5-6 minutes. Remove the chicken from the skillet and set aside.
3. In the same skillet, add the minced garlic and cook for about 1 minute until fragrant.
4. Sprinkle the flour over the garlic and stir well to create a roux. Cook for 2-3 minutes, or until the roux turns light golden brown.
5. Gradually whisk in the whole milk, chicken broth, and white wine (if using) until the sauce thickens and becomes smooth, about 5 minutes.
6. Stir in the grated Parmesan cheese and mozzarella cheese, and continue to cook until the cheese is melted and the sauce is creamy.
7. Return the cooked chicken to the skillet and add the cooked fettuccine pasta and broccoli. Toss everything together until well coated in the Alfredo sauce.
8. Season with salt and pepper, and garnish with fresh parsley.

**Nutritional Values:** Calories: 550 kcal | Fat: 20 g | Protein: 45 g | Carbs: 45 g | Net carbs: 40 g | Fiber: 5 g | Cholesterol: 150 mg | Sodium: 450 mg | Potassium: 500 mg

## Veggie-Packed Spaghetti Primavera

Serving: 4 | Prep time: 15 minutes | Cook time: 20 minutes

### Ingredients:

- 8 oz (225 g) whole wheat spaghetti
- 4 oz (115 g) cherry tomatoes, halved
- 4 oz (115 g) broccoli florets
- 4 oz (115 g) bell peppers, thinly sliced
- 4 oz (115 g) zucchini, thinly sliced
- 2 oz (60 g) red onion, thinly sliced
- 2 cloves garlic, minced
- 4 oz (115 g) baby spinach
- 2 oz (60 ml) olive oil
- 2 oz (60 g) grated Parmesan cheese
- 2 oz (60 ml) vegetable broth
- 1 oz (30 ml) white wine (optional)
- 1 tsp dried Italian herbs
- Salt and pepper to taste
- Fresh basil leaves, for garnish

### Directions:

1. Cook the whole wheat spaghetti according to package instructions until al dente. Drain and set aside.
2. In a large skillet, heat the olive oil over medium heat. Add the minced garlic and red onion, and sauté until they become translucent.
3. Add the cherry tomatoes, bell peppers, zucchini, and broccoli florets to the skillet. Cook for about 5 minutes until the vegetables are slightly tender.
4. Pour in the white wine (if using) and cook for 2 minutes to let the alcohol evaporate.
5. Stir in the vegetable broth, dried Italian herbs, and season with salt and pepper. Simmer for another 5 minutes.
6. Add the cooked whole wheat spaghetti and baby spinach to the skillet. Toss everything together until the spinach wilts and the pasta is coated with the vegetable mixture.
7. Serve the Spaghetti Primavera in individual plates, garnish with grated Parmesan cheese and fresh basil leaves.

**Nutritional Values:** Calories: 350 kcal | Fat: 14 g | Protein: 12 g | Carbs: 48 g | Net carbs: 40 g | Fiber: 8 g | Cholesterol: 5 mg | Sodium: 300 mg | Potassium: 450 mg



## Thai-Inspired Peanut Noodle Bowl

Serving: 4 | Prep time: 15 minutes | Cook time: 10 minutes

### Ingredients:

- 8 oz (225 g) rice noodles
- 4 oz (115 g) red bell pepper, thinly sliced
- 4 oz (115 g) cucumber, julienned
- 4 oz (115 g) carrots, julienned
- 4 oz (115 g) broccoli florets
- 4 oz (115 g) snow peas, trimmed and halved
- 4 oz (115 g) firm tofu, cubed
- 1 oz (30 ml) vegetable oil
- 2 cloves garlic, minced
- 2 oz (60 ml) soy sauce
- 2 oz (60 ml) lime juice
- 2 oz (60 g) peanut butter

- 1 oz (30 ml) honey
- 1 tsp grated fresh ginger
- 1/2 tsp red pepper flakes (adjust to taste)
- Chopped peanuts and fresh cilantro, for garnish

## Directions:

1. Cook the rice noodles according to the package instructions, then drain and rinse them under cold water. Set aside.
2. Heat vegetable oil in a large pan or wok over medium-high heat. Add the cubed tofu and stir-fry until it's golden and crispy. Remove tofu from the pan and set aside.
3. In the same pan, add minced garlic and cook for about 30 seconds until fragrant.
4. Add the red bell pepper, cucumber, carrots, broccoli, and snow peas to the pan. Stir-fry for about 3-5 minutes until the vegetables are tender-crisp.
5. In a small bowl, whisk together soy sauce, lime juice, peanut butter, honey, fresh ginger, and red pepper flakes until you have a smooth sauce.
6. Add the cooked rice noodles and tofu to the pan with the stir-fried vegetables. Pour the peanut sauce over the noodles and veggies.
7. Toss everything together until the noodles and vegetables are well coated with the sauce.
8. Serve the Peanut Noodle Bowl in individual bowls, garnish with chopped peanuts and fresh cilantro.

**Nutritional Values:** Calories: 400 kcal | Fat: 12 g | Protein: 10 g | Carbs: 65 g | Net carbs: 50 g | Fiber: 15 g | Cholesterol: 0 mg | Sodium: 800 mg | Potassium: 650 mg

**Useful Tip:** Adjust the red pepper flakes to control the spiciness level, and customize with your favorite veggies or protein. Enjoy the dish!

# Beef and Mushroom Stroganoff

Serving: 4 | Prep time: 15 minutes | Cook time: 20 minutes

## Ingredients:

- 12 oz (340 g) beef sirloin, thinly sliced
- 8 oz (225 g) cremini mushrooms, sliced
- 2 oz (60 ml) vegetable oil
- 1 oz (30 g) butter
- 1 small onion, finely chopped
- 2 cloves garlic, minced
- 2 oz (60 ml) beef broth
- 2 oz (60 ml) white wine
- 8 oz (225 g) sour cream
- 1 tsp Dijon mustard
- 1 tsp paprika
- Salt and pepper, to taste
- Fresh parsley, for garnish
- 10 oz (280 g) cooked egg noodles

## Directions:

1. In a large skillet, heat the vegetable oil over medium-high heat. Add the beef slices and cook until browned. Remove the beef from the skillet and set it aside.
2. In the same skillet, melt the butter and add the chopped onion. Sauté until the onion is soft and translucent.
3. Add the sliced mushrooms and minced garlic to the skillet. Cook until the mushrooms release their liquid and turn golden brown.
4. Pour in the white wine and beef broth, then stir to combine. Allow the mixture to simmer for a few minutes until it thickens slightly.

5. Stir in the sour cream, Dijon mustard, paprika, salt, and pepper. Mix well.
6. Return the cooked beef to the skillet and let it simmer for a few more minutes to heat through.
7. Serve the Beef and Mushroom Stroganoff over cooked egg noodles, garnished with fresh parsley.

**Nutritional Values:** Calories: 380 kcal | Fat: 24 g | Protein: 22 g | Carbs: 14 g | Net carbs: 12 g | Fiber: 2 g | Cholesterol: 85 mg | Sodium: 470 mg | Potassium: 450 mg

**Useful Tip:** For a creamier sauce, use full-fat sour cream, and adjust the seasoning to your taste. Enjoy the dish!

## Roasted Red Pepper and Spinach Fettuccine

Serving: 4 | Prep time: 15 minutes | Cook time: 20 minutes

**Ingredients:**

- 8 oz (225 g) fettuccine pasta
- 12 oz (340 g) roasted red peppers (from a jar), drained and chopped
- 6 oz (170 g) fresh spinach
- 2 oz (60 ml) olive oil
- 2 cloves garlic, minced
- 4 oz (115 g) heavy cream
- 2 oz (60 ml) vegetable broth
- 1 oz (30 g) grated Parmesan cheese
- Salt and black pepper, to taste
- Fresh basil leaves, for garnish

**Directions:**

1. Cook the fettuccine pasta according to the package instructions until al dente. Drain and set aside.
2. In a large skillet, heat the olive oil over medium heat. Add the minced garlic and cook until fragrant, about 1 minute.
3. Add the chopped roasted red peppers to the skillet and sauté for a couple of minutes.
4. Pour in the heavy cream and vegetable broth. Stir and bring to a gentle simmer.
5. Reduce the heat to low and stir in the grated Parmesan cheese. Continue stirring until the sauce thickens.
6. Add the fresh spinach to the skillet and cook just until wilted.
7. Season the sauce with salt and black pepper to taste.
8. Toss the cooked fettuccine pasta into the skillet and gently combine with the sauce.
9. Serve the Roasted Red Pepper and Spinach Fettuccine, garnished with fresh basil leaves.

**Nutritional Values:** Calories: 480 kcal | Fat: 28 g | Protein: 8 g | Carbs: 49 g | Net carbs: 43 g | Fiber: 6 g | Cholesterol: 60 mg | Sodium: 380 mg | Potassium: 400 mg

**Useful Tip:** You can adjust the thickness of the sauce by adding more or less heavy cream. Enjoy the dish!

## Mediterranean Orzo Salad

Serving: 4 | Prep time: 15 minutes | Cook time: 10 minutes

**Ingredients:**

- 8 oz (225 g) orzo pasta
- 2 oz (60 ml) olive oil
- 2 oz (60 ml) lemon juice
- 2 cloves garlic, minced
- 8 oz (225 g) cherry tomatoes, halved
- 4 oz (115 g) cucumber, diced
- 4 oz (115 g) Kalamata olives, pitted and sliced
- 4 oz (115 g) feta cheese, crumbled

- 2 oz (60 g) red onion, finely chopped
- 0,5 oz (15 g) fresh parsley, chopped
- Salt and black pepper, to taste

## Directions:

1. Cook the orzo pasta according to the package instructions until al dente. Drain and rinse with cold water to cool.
2. In a large mixing bowl, whisk together the olive oil, lemon juice, and minced garlic.
3. Add the cooked and cooled orzo pasta to the bowl and toss to coat with the dressing.
4. Gently fold in the halved cherry tomatoes, diced cucumber, sliced Kalamata olives, crumbled feta cheese, finely chopped red onion, and fresh parsley.
5. Season the salad with salt and black pepper to taste. Toss to combine all the ingredients.
6. Refrigerate the Mediterranean Orzo Salad for at least 30 minutes before serving to allow the flavors to meld.

**Nutritional Values:** Calories: 340 kcal | Fat: 16 g | Protein: 9 g | Carbs: 40 g | Net carbs: 36 g | Fiber: 4 g | Cholesterol: 25 mg | Sodium: 600 mg | Potassium: 340 mg

**Useful Tip:** You can customize this salad by adding other Mediterranean ingredients like artichoke hearts or roasted red peppers. Enjoy the dish!

# Creamy Sundried Tomato and Basil Farfalle

Serving: 4 | Prep time: 10 minutes | Cook time: 15 minutes

## Ingredients:

- 8 oz (225 g) farfalle pasta
- 2 oz (60 ml) olive oil
- 1 oz (30 g) sundried tomatoes, chopped
- 2 cloves garlic, minced
- 2 oz (60 ml) heavy cream
- 2 oz (60 ml) chicken broth
- 2 oz (60 ml) white wine
- 2 oz (60 ml) tomato sauce
- 0,5 oz (15 g) fresh basil, chopped
- Salt and black pepper, to taste
- Grated Parmesan cheese, for garnish

## Directions:

1. Cook the farfalle pasta according to the package instructions until al dente. Drain and set aside.
2. In a large skillet, heat the olive oil over medium heat. Add the chopped sundried tomatoes and minced garlic, and sauté for about 2 minutes until fragrant.
3. Pour in the heavy cream, chicken broth, and white wine. Simmer for 5 minutes, allowing the sauce to thicken slightly.
4. Stir in the tomato sauce and fresh basil. Continue to simmer for another 2-3 minutes, stirring frequently.
5. Season the sauce with salt and black pepper to taste.
6. Add the cooked farfalle pasta to the skillet, tossing it gently to coat with the creamy sundried tomato and basil sauce.
7. Garnish the dish with grated Parmesan cheese.

**Nutritional Values:** Calories: 470 kcal | Fat: 23 g | Protein: 9 g | Carbs: 54 g | Net carbs: 45 g | Fiber: 9 g | Cholesterol: 50 mg | Sodium: 650 mg | Potassium: 480 mg

**Useful Tip:** You can adjust the creaminess of the sauce by adding more or less heavy cream. Enjoy the dish!

# Turkey and Spinach Lasagna

Serving: 4 | Prep time: 20 minutes | Cook time: 40 minutes

Ingredients:

- 8 oz (225 g) lasagna noodles
- 12 oz (340 g) ground turkey
- 1 oz (30 ml) olive oil
- 1/2 onion, chopped
- 2 cloves garlic, minced
- 1 can (14 oz/400 g) crushed tomatoes
- 1 tsp tomato paste
- 1 tsp dried oregano
- 1 tsp dried basil
- Salt and black pepper, to taste
- 8 oz (225 g) fresh spinach
- 8 oz (225 g) ricotta cheese
- 4 oz (115 g) shredded mozzarella cheese
- 1 oz (30 g) grated Parmesan cheese
- Fresh basil leaves, for garnish

Directions:

1. Cook the lasagna noodles according to the package instructions until al dente. Drain, rinse with cold water, and set aside.
2. In a large skillet, heat the olive oil over medium heat. Add the chopped onion and minced garlic, and sauté until they become translucent.
3. Add the ground turkey and cook until browned, breaking it up with a spoon as it cooks.
4. Stir in the crushed tomatoes, tomato paste, dried oregano, and dried basil. Season with salt and black pepper. Simmer the turkey and tomato sauce for about 10 minutes.
5. Preheat your oven to 375°F (190°C).
6. In a separate skillet, wilt the fresh spinach over medium heat until it's cooked down, about 2-3 minutes. Drain any excess liquid.
7. In a large baking dish, layer the ingredients as follows: a small amount of the turkey and tomato sauce, a layer of lasagna noodles, half of the ricotta cheese, half of the spinach, and a portion of the shredded mozzarella. Repeat for a second layer.
8. Finish with a final layer of lasagna noodles, the remaining turkey and tomato sauce, and the rest of the mozzarella and Parmesan cheese.
9. Bake in the preheated oven for about 20 minutes or until the cheese is melted and bubbling.

Nutritional Values: Calories: 525 kcal | Fat: 21 g | Protein: 40 g | Carbs: 45 g | Net carbs: 40 g | Fiber: 5 g | Cholesterol: 95 mg | Sodium: 850 mg | Potassium: 740 mg

Useful Tip: You can add a touch of fresh basil leaves for a burst of flavor and garnish. Enjoy the dish!

# Spicy Cajun Shrimp Pasta

Serving: 4 | Prep Time: 15 minutes | Cook Time: 20 minutes

Ingredients:

- 12 oz (340 g) shrimp, peeled and deveined
- 8 oz (227 g) linguine or fettuccine pasta
- 3 tbsp olive oil
- 2 tbsp Cajun seasoning
- 1 red bell pepper, thinly sliced
- 1 green bell pepper, thinly sliced
- 1 small onion, finely chopped
- 3 cloves garlic, minced
- 14 oz (400 g) crushed tomatoes
- 8 oz (240 ml) heavy cream
- 2 oz (60 ml) chicken broth
- Salt and pepper to taste
- Fresh parsley, for garnish
- Grated Parmesan cheese, for serving

Directions:

1. Cook the pasta according to the package instructions until al dente, then drain and set aside.
2. In a large skillet, heat the olive oil over medium heat, add the shrimp, and sprinkle with 1 tbsp of Cajun seasoning. Cook the shrimp for 2-3 minutes on each side or until they turn pink. Remove the shrimp from the skillet and set them aside.
3. In the same skillet, add the sliced bell peppers, chopped onion, and garlic. Sauté for about 4-5 minutes or until the vegetables are tender.
4. Stir in the crushed tomatoes, heavy cream, chicken broth, and the remaining 1 tbsp of Cajun seasoning. Allow the sauce to simmer for 5-7 minutes, or until it thickens.
5. Return the cooked shrimp to the skillet, and let them heat through in the sauce. Season with salt and pepper to taste.
6. Serve the Cajun shrimp sauce over the cooked pasta, garnish with fresh parsley, and top with grated Parmesan cheese.

**Nutritional Values:** Calories: 450 kcal | Fat: 22 g | Protein: 25 g | Carbs: 40 g | Net Carbs: 36 g | Fiber: 4 g | Cholesterol: 200 mg | Sodium: 550 mg | Potassium: 800 mg

**Useful Tip:** For an extra kick of heat, add a pinch of red pepper flakes when you sauté the vegetables.

# Spinach and Ricotta Stuffed Shells

Serving: 4 | Prep Time: 20 minutes | Cook Time: 30 minutes

Ingredients:

- 8 oz (227 g) jumbo pasta shells
- 10 oz (283 g) frozen chopped spinach, thawed and squeezed dry
- 15 oz (425 g) ricotta cheese
- 4 oz (120 ml) marinara sauce
- 4 oz (120 ml) grated Parmesan cheese
- 4 oz (120 ml) shredded mozzarella cheese
- 1 egg
- 1 tsp garlic powder
- 1 tsp dried basil
- Salt and pepper to taste

Directions:

1. Preheat your oven to 350°F (175°C).

2. Cook the jumbo pasta shells according to the package instructions until they are al dente, then drain and set them aside.
3. In a mixing bowl, combine the thawed and squeezed dry chopped spinach, ricotta cheese, grated Parmesan cheese, egg, garlic powder, dried basil, salt, and pepper. Mix until well combined.
4. Fill each cooked pasta shell with the spinach and ricotta mixture and place them in a baking dish.
5. Pour the marinara sauce over the stuffed shells and top them with shredded mozzarella cheese.
6. Cover the baking dish with aluminum foil and bake for 20 minutes, then remove the foil and bake for an additional 10 minutes, or until the cheese is bubbly and golden.
7. Serve the Spinach and Ricotta Stuffed Shells hot and enjoy!

**Nutritional Values:** Calories: 400 kcal | Fat: 18 g | Protein: 25 g | Carbs: 32 g | Net Carbs: 26 g | Fiber: 6 g | Cholesterol: 100 mg | Sodium: 600 mg | Potassium: 500 mg

**Useful Tip:** If you have any leftover spinach and ricotta mixture, you can use it as a delicious filling for lasagna or as a dip for garlic bread.

# Pesto Tortellini Salad

Serving: 4 | Prep Time: 15 minutes | Cook Time: 10 minutes

## Ingredients:

- 9 oz (255 g) cheese tortellini
- 2 oz (60 ml) pesto sauce
- 2 oz (60 ml) extra virgin olive oil
- 2 oz (57 g) sun-dried tomatoes, chopped
- 2 oz (60 ml) grated Parmesan cheese
- 2 oz (57 g) baby spinach
- 2 oz (60 ml) pine nuts, toasted
- Salt and pepper to taste

## Directions:

1. Cook the cheese tortellini according to the package instructions until al dente, then drain and set them aside to cool.
2. In a large bowl, whisk together the pesto sauce and extra virgin olive oil to make the dressing.
3. Add the cooled tortellini, chopped sun-dried tomatoes, grated Parmesan cheese, and baby spinach to the bowl with the dressing. Toss to coat all the ingredients evenly.
4. Season the salad with salt and pepper to taste and sprinkle toasted pine nuts on top.
5. Chill the Pesto Tortellini Salad in the refrigerator for about 30 minutes before serving.

**Nutritional Values:** Calories: 420 kcal | Fat: 28 g | Protein: 12 g | Carbs: 32 g | Net Carbs: 28 g | Fiber: 4 g | Cholesterol: 10 mg | Sodium: 380 mg | Potassium: 300 mg

**Useful Tip:** To toast pine nuts, simply place them in a dry skillet over medium heat and stir frequently until they turn golden brown. Be careful not to overcook them as they can burn quickly.

# Beef and Vegetable Lo Mein

Serving: 4 | Prep Time: 15 minutes | Cook Time: 20 minutes

**Ingredients:**

- 8 oz (227 g) lo mein noodles
- 8 oz (227 g) flank steak, thinly sliced
- 2 tbsp vegetable oil
- 2 cloves garlic, minced
- 1 tsp fresh ginger, minced
- 1 red bell pepper, thinly sliced
- 6 oz (175 g) broccoli florets
- 1 carrot, julienned
- 4 oz (120 ml) low-sodium soy sauce
- 2 tbsp oyster sauce
- 1 tsp sesame oil
- 2 green onions, sliced
- Sesame seeds for garnish (optional)

**Directions:**

1. Cook the lo mein noodles according to the package instructions, then drain and set aside.
2. In a large skillet, heat 1 tablespoon of vegetable oil over medium-high heat. Add the thinly sliced flank steak and stir-fry for about 2-3 minutes until it's browned. Remove the beef from the skillet and set it aside.
3. In the same skillet, add the remaining 1 tablespoon of vegetable oil. Stir in the minced garlic and ginger, and sauté for about 30 seconds until fragrant.
4. Add the red bell pepper, broccoli florets, and julienned carrot to the skillet. Stir-fry the vegetables for 3-4 minutes until they are tender-crisp.
5. Return the cooked beef to the skillet, and add the cooked lo mein noodles, low-sodium soy sauce, oyster sauce, and sesame oil. Toss everything together to combine and heat through.
6. Garnish the Beef and Vegetable Lo Mein with sliced green onions and sesame seeds (if desired).

**Nutritional Values:** Calories: 380 kcal | Fat: 12 g | Protein: 22 g | Carbs: 45 g | Net Carbs: 37 g | Fiber: 8 g | Cholesterol: 45 mg | Sodium: 850 mg | Potassium: 600 mg

**Useful Tip:** If you prefer a spicier flavor, you can add a pinch of red pepper flakes or a drizzle of sriracha sauce when you toss everything together.

# Lemon Herb Chicken and Capellini

Serving: 4 | Prep Time: 15 minutes | Cook Time: 20 minutes

**Ingredients:**

- 8 oz (227 g) capellini (angel hair) pasta
- 4 boneless, skinless chicken breasts (4 oz each, 113 g)
- 2 tbsp olive oil
- 2 cloves garlic, minced
- Zest of 1 lemon
- Juice of 1 lemon
- 2 tbsp white wine
- 2 tbsp chicken broth
- 1 tsp dried thyme
- 1 tsp dried rosemary
- Salt and pepper to taste
- Fresh parsley, for garnish
- Lemon slices, for garnish

**Directions:**

1. Cook the capellini pasta according to the package instructions until al dente, then drain and set aside.

2. Season the chicken breasts with dried thyme, dried rosemary, salt, and pepper.

3. In a large skillet, heat the olive oil over medium-high heat. Add the seasoned chicken breasts and cook for about 6-8 minutes on each side or until they are cooked through and have a golden brown crust.

4. Remove the chicken from the skillet and set it aside.

5. In the same skillet, add the minced garlic and sauté for about 30 seconds until fragrant.

6. Add the lemon zest, lemon juice, white wine, and chicken broth to the skillet. Stir to combine and simmer for 2-3 minutes to create a flavorful sauce.

7. Return the cooked capellini to the skillet and toss it in the lemon herb sauce until well-coated.

8. Serve the Lemon Herb Chicken and Capellini topped with the cooked chicken breasts, fresh parsley, and lemon slices.

**Nutritional Values:** Calories: 360 kcal | Fat: 8 g | Protein: 28 g | Carbs: 45 g | Net Carbs: 41 g | Fiber: 4 g | Cholesterol: 70 mg | Sodium: 320 mg | Potassium: 450 mg

**Useful Tip:** For extra freshness, you can add a handful of sautéed asparagus or cherry tomatoes to the dish for added color and flavor.

# Greek Salad with Tzatziki Dressing

Serving: 4 | Prep Time: 15 minutes | Cook Time: 0 minutes

**Ingredients:**

- 8 oz (227 g) cucumbers, diced
- 8 oz (227 g) tomatoes, diced
- 4 oz (113 g) red onion, finely chopped
- 4 oz (113 g) Kalamata olives, pitted and halved
- 4 oz (113 g) feta cheese, crumbled
- 4 oz (113 g) green bell pepper, diced
- 2 oz (60 ml) extra virgin olive oil
- 2 tbsp red wine vinegar
- 1 tsp dried oregano
- Salt and pepper to taste
- Fresh parsley, for garnish
- Lemon wedges, for serving

**For the Tzatziki Dressing:**

- 4 oz (120 ml) Greek yogurt
- 1/2 cucumber, grated and squeezed dry
- 2 cloves garlic, minced
- 1 tbsp fresh lemon juice
- 1 tbsp fresh dill, chopped
- Salt and pepper to taste

**Directions:**

1. In a large salad bowl, combine the diced cucumbers, tomatoes, red onion, Kalamata olives, feta cheese, and green bell pepper.

2. In a separate bowl, whisk together the extra virgin olive oil, red wine vinegar, dried oregano, salt, and pepper to make the salad dressing. Pour this dressing over the salad ingredients and toss to coat evenly.

3. In another bowl, prepare the Tzatziki dressing by combining Greek yogurt, grated and squeezed dry cucumber, minced garlic, fresh lemon juice, fresh dill, salt, and pepper.

4. Serve the Greek Salad with a dollop of Tzatziki dressing on top, garnished with fresh parsley, and lemon wedges on the side.

**Nutritional Values:** Calories: 350 kcal | Fat: 25 g | Protein: 9 g | Carbs: 23 g | Net Carbs: 15 g | Fiber: 8 g | Cholesterol: 20 mg | Sodium: 700 mg | Potassium: 550 mg

**Useful Tip:** To enhance the flavors, let the salad chill in the refrigerator for about 30 minutes before serving.

## Tuna and White Bean Salad

Serving: 4 | Prep time: 15 minutes | Cook time: 0 minutes

**Ingredients:**

- 12 oz (340 g) canned tuna, drained
- 12 oz (340 g) canned white beans, drained and rinsed
- 4 oz (113 g) red onion, finely chopped
- 4 oz (113 g) celery, finely chopped
- 2 oz (57 g) fresh parsley, chopped
- 2 oz (57 g) olive oil
- 2 oz (57 g) lemon juice
- 1 oz (28 g) Dijon mustard
- Salt and pepper to taste

**Directions:**

1. In a large bowl, combine the drained tuna, white beans, finely chopped red onion, celery, and fresh parsley.
2. In a separate small bowl, whisk together the olive oil, lemon juice, and Dijon mustard until well combined.
3. Pour the dressing over the tuna and white bean mixture and gently toss to coat all the ingredients.
4. Season the salad with salt and pepper to taste. Adjust the seasoning as needed.
5. Allow the salad to marinate in the refrigerator for at least 30 minutes before serving to let the flavors meld together.

**Nutritional Values:** Calories: 320 kcal | Fat: 14 g | Protein: 31 g | Carbs: 20 g | Net carbs: 14 g | Fiber: 6 g | Cholesterol: 42 mg | Sodium: 610 mg | Potassium: 690 mg

**Useful Tip:** This salad is even better the next day, so consider making it in advance for a quick and healthy meal.

## Chickpea and Cucumber Salad

Serving: 4 | Prep time: 15 minutes | Cook time: 0 minutes

**Ingredients:**

- 8 oz (227 g) canned chickpeas, drained and rinsed
- 8 oz (227 g) cucumber, diced
- 2 oz (57 g) red bell pepper, finely chopped
- 2 oz (57 g) red onion, finely chopped
- 2 oz (57 g) fresh parsley, chopped
- 1 oz (28 g) lemon juice
- 1 oz (28 g) extra-virgin olive oil
- 1 oz (28 g) red wine vinegar
- Salt and pepper to taste

**Directions:**

1. In a large salad bowl, combine the drained and rinsed chickpeas, diced cucumber, finely chopped red bell pepper, finely chopped red onion, and fresh parsley.
2. In a separate bowl, whisk together the lemon juice, extra-virgin olive oil, red wine vinegar, salt, and pepper to create the dressing.
3. Pour the dressing over the chickpea and vegetable mixture.
4. Gently toss the salad to ensure the dressing evenly coats all the ingredients.

**Nutritional Values:** Calories: 190 kcal | Fat: 10 g | Protein: 5 g | Carbs: 20 g | Net carbs: 13 g | Fiber: 7 g | Cholesterol: 0 mg | Sodium: 280 mg | Potassium: 290 mg

## Caprese Salad

Serving: 4 | Prep Time: 10 minutes | Cook Time: 0 minutes

Ingredients:

- 8 oz (227 g) fresh mozzarella, sliced
- 8 oz (227 g) ripe tomatoes, sliced
- 2 oz (57 g) fresh basil leaves
- 2 tbsp extra virgin olive oil
- 2 tbsp balsamic glaze
- Salt and pepper to taste

Directions:

1. Arrange the fresh mozzarella slices, tomato slices, and fresh basil leaves on a serving platter.
2. Drizzle extra virgin olive oil and balsamic glaze over the salad.
3. Season with salt and pepper to taste.

Nutritional Values: Calories: 260 kcal | Fat: 20 g | Protein: 14 g | Carbs: 6 g | Net Carbs: 4 g | Fiber: 2 g | Cholesterol: 45 mg | Sodium: 300 mg | Potassium: 300 mg

Useful Tip: For a twist on the classic Caprese, you can add a drizzle of honey for a touch of sweetness or a sprinkle of toasted pine nuts for a delightful crunch.

## Egg Salad with Greens

Serving: 4 | Prep time: 10 minutes | Cook time: 10 minutes

Ingredients:

- 8 large eggs
- 4 oz (113 g) mixed greens (e.g., spinach, arugula, and kale)
- 1 oz (28 g) cherry tomatoes, halved
- 1 oz (28 g) cucumber, sliced
- 1 oz (28 g) red bell pepper, diced
- 1 oz (28 g) red onion, finely chopped
- 2 oz (57 ml) Greek yogurt
- 1 oz (28 ml) olive oil
- 1 oz (28 ml) lemon juice
- 1 tsp Dijon mustard
- Salt and pepper to taste
- 1/2 tsp dried dill (optional)
- Fresh chives for garnish (optional)

Directions:

1. Place the eggs in a saucepan and cover them with water. Bring the water to a boil, then reduce the heat to a simmer and cook for 9-12 minutes, depending on your desired yolk consistency (9 minutes for soft-boiled, 12 minutes for hard-boiled).
2. While the eggs are cooking, prepare an ice bath by filling a large bowl with ice and cold water. When the eggs are done, immediately transfer them to the ice bath to cool for a few minutes. This helps in easy peeling.
3. Once the eggs are cooled, peel and chop them into bite-sized pieces.
4. In a large salad bowl, combine the mixed greens, cherry tomatoes, cucumber, red bell pepper, and red onion.
5. In a separate bowl, whisk together the Greek yogurt, olive oil, lemon juice, Dijon mustard, salt, and pepper to create the dressing. Add dried dill for extra flavor if desired.
6. Add the chopped eggs to the salad bowl and drizzle the dressing over the salad. Toss gently to coat all the ingredients with the dressing.

7.  Garnish with fresh chives if desired.

**Nutritional Values:** Calories: 240 kcal | Fat: 18 g | Protein: 13 g | Carbs: 7 g | Net carbs: 5 g | Fiber: 2 g | Cholesterol: 380 mg | Sodium: 250 mg | Potassium: 320 mg

**Useful Tip:** To make peeling the eggs even easier, you can add a teaspoon of vinegar to the boiling water.

# SNACKS AND SANDWICHES

## Crispy Roasted Chickpeas

Serving: 4 | Prep Time: 10 minutes | Cook Time: 35 minutes

**Ingredients:**

- 15 oz (425 g) canned chickpeas, drained and rinsed
- 2 tbsp olive oil
- 1 tsp smoked paprika
- 1/2 tsp cumin
- 1/2 tsp garlic powder
- 1/2 tsp onion powder
- Salt and pepper to taste

**Directions:**

1. Preheat your oven to 400°F (200°C).
2. After draining and rinsing the chickpeas, pat them dry with a paper towel to remove excess moisture.
3. In a bowl, combine the chickpeas, olive oil, smoked paprika, cumin, garlic powder, onion powder, salt, and pepper. Toss until the chickpeas are evenly coated with the seasonings.
4. Spread the seasoned chickpeas in a single layer on a baking sheet.
5. Roast in the preheated oven for 30-35 minutes, or until the chickpeas are golden brown and crispy, shaking the pan or stirring the chickpeas occasionally for even cooking.
6. Remove the roasted chickpeas from the oven, let them cool slightly, and serve.

**Nutritional Values:** Calories: 150 kcal | Fat: 6 g | Protein: 5 g | Carbs: 20 g | Net Carbs: 13 g | Fiber: 7 g | Cholesterol: 0 mg | Sodium: 300 mg | Potassium: 190 mg

**Useful Tip:** You can customize the flavors by experimenting with different seasonings like chili powder, curry, or a touch of lemon zest for variety.

## Spicy Buffalo Cauliflower Bites

Serving: 4 | Prep Time: 15 minutes | Cook Time: 25 minutes

**Ingredients:**

- 16 oz (454 g) cauliflower florets
- 2 tbsp olive oil
- 4 oz (120 ml) hot sauce (adjust to taste)
- 2 tbsp melted butter
- 1 tsp garlic powder
- 1 tsp onion powder
- 0.5 tsp paprika
- 0.5 tsp salt
- 0.25 tsp black pepper
- Ranch or blue cheese dressing for dipping (optional)

**Directions:**

1. Preheat your oven to 450°F (230°C) and line a baking sheet with parchment paper.
2. In a large bowl, toss the cauliflower florets with olive oil, garlic powder, onion powder, paprika, salt, and black pepper until they are evenly coated.

3. Spread the seasoned cauliflower on the prepared baking sheet and roast in the preheated oven for 20-25 minutes, or until the florets are tender and start to turn golden brown.
4. While the cauliflower is roasting, in a separate bowl, mix the hot sauce and melted butter to make the spicy Buffalo sauce.
5. Remove the cauliflower from the oven and drizzle the Buffalo sauce over the roasted florets, ensuring they are well coated. Return the cauliflower to the oven and bake for an additional 5 minutes.
6. Serve the Spicy Buffalo Cauliflower Bites with your choice of dipping sauce, such as ranch or blue cheese.

**Nutritional Values:** Calories: 150 kcal | Fat: 11 g | Protein: 2 g | Carbs: 10 g | Net Carbs: 8 g | Fiber: 2 g | Cholesterol: 20 mg | Sodium: 1000 mg | Potassium: 350 mg

**Useful Tip:** For extra crispiness, you can lightly coat the cauliflower florets with a thin layer of cornstarch before tossing them in the seasonings.

# Avocado and Black Bean Salsa

Serving: 4 | Prep Time: 15 minutes | Cook Time: 0 minutes

## Ingredients:

- 8 oz (227 g) canned black beans, drained and rinsed
- 2 ripe avocados, diced
- 4 oz (113 g) cherry tomatoes, quartered
- 2 oz (57 g) red onion, finely chopped
- 2 oz (57 g) fresh cilantro, chopped
- 2 oz (57 g) corn kernels (canned or frozen, thawed)
- 1 jalapeño pepper, seeds removed and finely diced (adjust to taste)
- Juice of 2 limes
- 2 tbsp olive oil
- 1 tsp cumin
- Salt and pepper to taste
- Tortilla chips for serving

## Directions:

1. In a large bowl, combine the black beans, diced avocados, quartered cherry tomatoes, finely chopped red onion, chopped cilantro, corn kernels, and finely diced jalapeño pepper.
2. In a small bowl, whisk together the lime juice, olive oil, cumin, salt, and pepper to create the dressing.
3. Pour the dressing over the avocado and black bean mixture, gently toss to combine, and ensure everything is well coated.
4. Serve the Avocado and Black Bean Salsa with tortilla chips for dipping.

**Nutritional Values:** Calories: 220 kcal | Fat: 12 g | Protein: 5 g | Carbs: 25 g | Net Carbs: 17 g | Fiber: 8 g | Cholesterol: 0 mg | Sodium: 300 mg | Potassium: 700 mg

**Useful Tip:** To prevent the avocados from browning, add a little extra lime juice or keep the avocado pits in the salsa until serving.

# Turkey and Avocado Roll-Ups

Serving: 4 | Prep Time: 10 minutes | Cook Time: 0 minutes

Ingredients:

- 8 oz (227 g) deli turkey slices
- 2 ripe avocados, sliced
- 4 oz (113 g) cream cheese, softened
- 2 oz (57 g) baby spinach leaves
- 1 oz (28 g) sun-dried tomatoes, thinly sliced
- 1 tbsp olive oil
- 1 tbsp balsamic glaze
- Salt and pepper to taste

Directions:

1. Lay out the turkey slices on a clean surface.
2. Spread a thin layer of softened cream cheese over each turkey slice.
3. Arrange avocado slices, baby spinach leaves, and sun-dried tomatoes evenly over the cream cheese layer.
4. Season with salt and pepper to taste.
5. Roll up the turkey slices tightly, starting from one end, to form the roll-ups.
6. Drizzle olive oil and balsamic glaze over the top of the roll-ups.
7. Secure with toothpicks, if necessary, and slice each roll-up into bite-sized pieces.
8. Serve the Turkey and Avocado Roll-Ups chilled.

Nutritional Values: Calories: 280 kcal | Fat: 21 g | Protein: 16 g | Carbs: 8 g | Net Carbs: 3 g | Fiber: 5 g | Cholesterol: 60 mg | Sodium: 450 mg | Potassium: 580 mg

Useful Tip: To prevent the avocado from browning, sprinkle a little lemon juice over the avocado slices before assembling the roll-ups.

# Spiced Roasted Edamame

Serving: 4 | Prep Time: 10 minutes | Cook Time: 20 minutes

Ingredients:

- 16 oz (454 g) frozen edamame, thawed
- 1 tbsp olive oil
- 1 tsp smoked paprika
- 1/2 tsp cumin
- 1/2 tsp garlic powder
- 1/4 tsp cayenne pepper (adjust to taste)
- Salt and pepper to taste
- 1 tbsp grated Parmesan cheese (optional)

Directions:

1. Preheat your oven to 375°F (190°C) and line a baking sheet with parchment paper.
2. In a bowl, toss the thawed edamame with olive oil, smoked paprika, cumin, garlic powder, cayenne pepper, salt, and pepper until they are evenly coated with the seasonings.
3. Spread the seasoned edamame in a single layer on the prepared baking sheet.
4. Roast in the preheated oven for 20 minutes, or until the edamame is crisp and lightly browned, stirring them halfway through for even cooking.
5. If desired, sprinkle the roasted edamame with grated Parmesan cheese while they are still hot from the oven.
6. Serve the Spiced Roasted Edamame as a crunchy and flavorful snack.

**Nutritional Values:** Calories: 150 kcal | Fat: 8 g | Protein: 12 g | Carbs: 10 g | Net Carbs: 4 g | Fiber: 6 g | Cholesterol: 0 mg | Sodium: 300 mg | Potassium: 400 mg

**Useful Tip:** You can customize the spice level by adjusting the amount of cayenne pepper to suit your taste preferences.

## Nut Butter and Banana Sandwich

Serving: 4 | Prep Time: 5 minutes | Cook Time: 0 minutes

### Ingredients:

- 8 slices whole-grain bread (about 16 oz or 454 g)
- 8 tbsp nut butter (such as almond, peanut, or cashew butter)
- 2 ripe bananas, thinly sliced (about 10 oz or 283 g)
- 1 tbsp honey or maple syrup (optional)
- Cinnamon, to taste
- Chia seeds, for garnish (optional)

### Directions:

1. Lay out the 8 slices of whole-grain bread on a clean surface.
2. Spread 1 tbsp (15 ml) of your chosen nut butter onto 4 of the bread slices.
3. Arrange the thinly sliced bananas evenly over the nut butter.
4. If desired, drizzle a touch of honey or maple syrup over the banana slices for added sweetness.
5. Sprinkle a pinch of cinnamon on top of the bananas for extra flavor.
6. Close the sandwiches by placing the remaining 4 slices of bread on top.
7. Optionally, sprinkle some chia seeds over the sandwich for added crunch and nutrition.
8. Slice the sandwiches in half, if preferred, and serve.

**Nutritional Values:** Calories: 350 kcal | Fat: 15 g | Protein: 9 g | Carbs: 48 g | Net Carbs: 33 g | Fiber: 15 g | Cholesterol: 0 mg | Sodium: 300 mg | Potassium: 570 mg

**Useful Tip:** For a healthier option, you can use whole-grain or whole wheat bread and choose natural nut butters without added sugars or oils.

## Quinoa and Black Bean Stuffed Peppers

Serving: 4 | Prep Time: 15 minutes | Cook Time: 40 minutes

### Ingredients:

- 4 large bell peppers, any color (about 28 oz or 794 g)
- 6.5 oz (184 g) quinoa
- 15 oz (425 g) canned black beans, drained and rinsed
- 4 oz (113 g) shredded cheddar cheese
- 4 oz (113 g) corn kernels (canned or frozen, thawed)
- 1 tsp cumin
- 1/2 tsp chili powder
- 1/2 tsp garlic powder
- Salt and pepper to taste
- 16 oz (473 ml) tomato sauce

1. Preheat your oven to 375°F (190°C).
2. Cut the tops off the bell peppers and remove the seeds and membranes. Set aside.
3. In a saucepan, combine the quinoa with 2 cups (473 ml) of water. Bring to a boil, reduce the heat, cover, and simmer for 15 minutes or until the quinoa is cooked and the water is absorbed. Fluff with a fork.
4. In a large mixing bowl, combine the cooked quinoa, black beans, half of the shredded cheddar cheese, corn kernels, cumin, chili powder, garlic powder, salt, and pepper.
5. Stuff each bell pepper with the quinoa and black bean mixture, pressing it down gently to pack the peppers.
6. Place the stuffed peppers in a baking dish and pour the tomato sauce over them.
7. Cover the dish with aluminum foil and bake in the preheated oven for 30-35 minutes, or until the peppers are tender.
8. Remove the foil, sprinkle the remaining cheddar cheese over the stuffed peppers, and bake for an additional 5 minutes or until the cheese is melted and bubbly.
9. Serve the Quinoa and Black Bean Stuffed Peppers with extra tomato sauce if desired.

**Nutritional Values:** Calories: 450 kcal | Fat: 10 g | Protein: 17 g | Carbs: 72 g | Net Carbs: 60 g | Fiber: 12 g | Cholesterol: 25 mg | Sodium: 900 mg | Potassium: 1000 mg

**Useful Tip:** You can customize this dish by adding your favorite toppings like sour cream, guacamole, or fresh cilantro.

## Cottage Cheese with Pineapple and Walnuts

Serving: 4 | Prep Time: 10 minutes | Cook Time: 0 minutes

Ingredients:

- 16 oz (454 g) low-fat cottage cheese
- 8 oz (227 g) canned pineapple chunks, drained
- 2 oz (57 g) walnuts, chopped
- 1 tbsp honey
- 1 tsp vanilla extract
- 1/2 tsp ground cinnamon

Directions:

1. In a large bowl, combine the low-fat cottage cheese, drained pineapple chunks, and chopped walnuts.
2. Drizzle honey and vanilla extract over the mixture.
3. Sprinkle ground cinnamon on top for extra flavor.
4. Gently fold all the ingredients together until well combined.
5. Chill the Cottage Cheese with Pineapple and Walnuts in the refrigerator for at least 15 minutes before serving.

**Nutritional Values:** Calories: 220 kcal | Fat: 8 g | Protein: 20 g | Carbs: 18 g | Net Carbs: 14 g | Fiber: 4 g | Cholesterol: 10 mg | Sodium: 500 mg | Potassium: 250 mg

**Useful Tip:** For added freshness, you can use fresh pineapple chunks instead of canned, and adjust the honey to your desired sweetness level.

# Smoked Salmon Cucumber Bites

Serving: 4 | Prep Time: 15 minutes | Cook Time: 0 minutes

Ingredients:

- 4 oz (113 g) smoked salmon
- 2 large cucumbers
- 4 oz (113 g) cream cheese
- 2 tbsp fresh dill, finely chopped
- 1 lemon, zested
- Salt and pepper, to taste

Directions:

1. Wash and peel the cucumbers, leaving some strips of skin for a decorative touch. Slice the cucumbers into rounds, about 1/2 inch thick.
2. In a small bowl, combine the cream cheese, fresh dill, lemon zest, salt, and pepper. Mix until all the ingredients are well incorporated.
3. Spread a generous amount of the cream cheese mixture on each cucumber round.
4. Carefully tear the smoked salmon into smaller pieces and place them on top of the cream cheese layer.
5. Garnish with additional fresh dill and a little extra lemon zest for a burst of flavor.
6. Serve the Smoked Salmon Cucumber Bites as an elegant and delicious appetizer.

Nutritional Values: Calories: 140 kcal | Fat: 9 g | Protein: 9 g | Carbs: 6 g | Net Carbs: 4 g | Fiber: 2 g | Cholesterol: 30 mg | Sodium: 480 mg | Potassium: 350 mg

Useful Tip: To add an extra kick of flavor, you can sprinkle a bit of capers on top of the smoked salmon before serving.

# Almond and Coconut Energy Bites

Serving: 4 | Prep Time: 15 minutes | Cook Time: 0 minutes

Ingredients:

- 4 oz (113 g) almonds
- 2 oz (57 g) dried dates
- 2 oz (57 g) shredded coconut
- 1 oz (28 g) almond butter
- 1 tbsp honey
- 1 tsp vanilla extract
- 1/2 tsp cinnamon
- Pinch of salt

Directions:

1. In a food processor, combine the almonds, dried dates, shredded coconut, almond butter, honey, vanilla extract, cinnamon, and a pinch of salt.
2. Pulse the mixture until it forms a sticky and crumbly texture, ensuring that the ingredients are well combined.
3. Using your hands, scoop out small portions of the mixture and roll them into bite-sized balls.
4. Place the Almond and Coconut Energy Bites on a parchment paper-lined tray or plate and refrigerate for at least 30 minutes to help them set.
5. Once chilled and firm, transfer the energy bites to an airtight container and store them in the refrigerator.
6. These energy bites make for a convenient and nutritious on-the-go snack.

Nutritional Values: Calories: 230 kcal | Fat: 15 g | Protein: 6 g | Carbs: 21 g | Net Carbs: 15 g | Fiber: 6 g | Cholesterol: 0 mg | Sodium: 60 mg | Potassium: 260 mg

Useful Tip: Customize your energy bites by adding dark chocolate chips, chia seeds, or a sprinkle of cocoa powder for variety.

## Caprese Skewers with Balsamic Glaze

Serving: 4 | Prep Time: 20 minutes | Cook Time: 5 minutes

**Ingredients:**

- 8 oz (227 g) fresh mozzarella balls
- 2 oz (57 g) cherry tomatoes
- 1 oz (28 g) fresh basil leaves
- 2 oz (57 ml) balsamic vinegar
- 1 oz (28 ml) extra virgin olive oil
- 1 clove garlic, minced
- Salt and pepper, to taste
- Wooden skewers

**Directions:**

1. In a small saucepan, combine balsamic vinegar and minced garlic. Simmer over low heat for about 5 minutes until the mixture thickens and reduces by half. Set aside to cool.
2. Thread a mozzarella ball, a cherry tomato, and a fresh basil leaf onto each wooden skewer. Repeat until all the skewers are assembled.
3. Arrange the Caprese skewers on a serving platter.
4. Drizzle extra virgin olive oil and the balsamic glaze over the skewers.
5. Season with salt and pepper to taste.
6. These Caprese Skewers with Balsamic Glaze make a delightful appetizer for any occasion.

**Nutritional Values:** Calories: 190 kcal | Fat: 14 g | Protein: 8 g | Carbs: 8 g | Net Carbs: 7 g | Fiber: 1 g | Cholesterol: 25 mg | Sodium: 200 mg | Potassium: 120 mg

**Useful Tip:** Soak the wooden skewers in water for about 30 minutes before assembling the Caprese skewers to prevent them from splintering.

## Turkey and Cranberry Panini

Serving: 4 | Prep Time: 10 minutes | Cook Time: 5 minutes

**Ingredients:**

- 8 slices of whole grain bread (16 oz / 454 g)
- 8 oz (227 g) sliced turkey breast
- 4 oz (113 g) cranberry sauce
- 4 oz (113 g) baby spinach
- 4 oz (113 g) Swiss cheese, thinly sliced
- 1 oz (28 ml) olive oil
- 1 tsp Dijon mustard
- Salt and pepper to taste

**Directions:**

1. Preheat a panini press or a grill pan.
2. In a small bowl, mix the olive oil and Dijon mustard. Brush one side of each slice of bread with this mixture.
3. Lay the bread slices, oil-side down, on a clean surface.
4. On half of the bread slices, layer the turkey, cranberry sauce, baby spinach, and Swiss cheese. Season with a pinch of salt and pepper.
5. Top with the remaining bread slices, oil-side up, to create sandwiches.

6. Place the sandwiches in the preheated panini press or grill pan and cook for about 4-5 minutes or until the bread is toasted, and the cheese is melted.

7. Slice the Turkey and Cranberry Panini in half, serve, and enjoy this delicious sandwich.

**Nutritional Values:** Calories: 420 kcal | Fat: 16 g | Protein: 24 g | Carbs: 45 g | Net Carbs: 34 g | Fiber: 11 g | Cholesterol: 45 mg | Sodium: 680 mg | Potassium: 400 mg

**Useful Tip:** Don't have a panini press? You can use a regular skillet and press the sandwich down with a heavy pan or a clean brick wrapped in foil.

## Roast Beef and Horseradish Sandwich

Serving: 4 | Prep Time: 10 minutes | Cook Time: 0 minutes

### Ingredients:

- 8 slices of whole grain bread (16 oz / 454 g)
- 8 oz (227 g) thinly sliced roast beef
- 4 oz (113 g) horseradish sauce
- 4 oz (113 g) arugula
- 4 oz (113 g) red onion, thinly sliced
- 4 oz (113 g) provolone cheese, thinly sliced
- Salt and black pepper to taste

### Directions:

1. Lay out the 8 slices of whole grain bread on a clean surface.
2. On 4 of the bread slices, spread a generous layer of horseradish sauce.
3. Top the horseradish sauce with roast beef, provolone cheese, arugula, and red onion.
4. Season with a pinch of salt and black pepper.
5. Place the remaining 4 slices of bread on top to create sandwiches.
6. Slice the Roast Beef and Horseradish Sandwiches in half and serve.

**Nutritional Values:** Calories: 380 kcal | Fat: 14 g | Protein: 30 g | Carbs: 38 g | Net Carbs: 29 g | Fiber: 9 g | Cholesterol: 60 mg | Sodium: 860 mg | Potassium: 470 mg

**Useful Tip:** If you like your sandwich toasted, you can use a panini press or a skillet to achieve that golden, crispy texture.

## BBQ Pulled Chicken Slider

Serving: 4 | Prep Time: 15 minutes | Cook Time: 30 minutes

### Ingredients:

- 16 oz (454 g) boneless, skinless chicken breasts
- 4 oz (113 g) BBQ sauce
- 4 whole wheat slider buns (about 2 oz / 56 g each)
- 4 oz (113 g) coleslaw
- 2 oz (57 g) dill pickles, sliced
- 1 oz (28 g) red onion, thinly sliced
- 1 tsp olive oil
- Salt and black pepper to taste

### Directions:

1. Season the chicken breasts with salt and black pepper.
2. Heat olive oil in a skillet over medium-high heat.

3. Cook the chicken breasts for about 5-7 minutes on each side, or until they are cooked through and have a nice sear.
4. While the chicken is cooking, toast the slider buns in a toaster or oven until they are slightly crispy.
5. Remove the cooked chicken from the skillet, shred it using two forks, and mix it with BBQ sauce.
6. Assemble the sliders by placing a portion of BBQ pulled chicken on the bottom half of each bun.
7. Top with coleslaw, dill pickles, and red onion slices.
8. Place the top half of the bun on the ingredients to form the sliders.

**Nutritional Values:** Calories: 330 kcal | Fat: 7 g | Protein: 31 g | Carbs: 32 g | Net Carbs: 25 g | Fiber: 7 g | Cholesterol: 75 mg | Sodium: 660 mg | Potassium: 610 mg

**Useful Tip:** For a smokier flavor, you can grill the chicken breasts instead of cooking them in a skillet.

# Grilled Tofu and Vegetable Pita

Serving: 4 | Prep Time: 20 minutes | Cook Time: 15 minutes

**Ingredients:**

- 12 oz (340 g) extra-firm tofu, sliced into 1/2-inch strips
- 8 oz (227 g) bell peppers (mixed colors), sliced into strips
- 8 oz (227 g) zucchini, sliced into rounds
- 4 oz (113 g) red onion, thinly sliced
- 4 whole wheat pita bread pockets
- 2 oz (57 g) hummus
- 1 oz (28 g) baby spinach leaves
- 1 tsp olive oil
- 1 tsp lemon juice
- 1/2 tsp dried oregano
- Salt and black pepper to taste

**Directions:**

1. Preheat a grill or grill pan over medium-high heat.
2. In a bowl, mix the olive oil, lemon juice, dried oregano, salt, and black pepper.
3. Brush the tofu slices, bell peppers, zucchini, and red onion with the olive oil mixture.
4. Grill the tofu for about 2-3 minutes on each side until grill marks appear. Remove and set aside.
5. Grill the bell peppers, zucchini, and red onion until they are tender and slightly charred, about 3-4 minutes per side.
6. While the vegetables are grilling, warm the whole wheat pita bread pockets on the grill for 1-2 minutes on each side.
7. To assemble the pita, spread 1/2 oz (14 g) of hummus inside each pita pocket.
8. Place the grilled tofu, mixed grilled vegetables, and a handful of baby spinach inside each pita.
9. Serve immediately.

**Nutritional Values:** Calories: 320 kcal | Fat: 11 g | Protein: 16 g | Carbs: 40 g | Net Carbs: 29 g | Fiber: 11 g | Cholesterol: 0 mg | Sodium: 480 mg | Potassium: 370 mg

**Useful Tip:** For added flavor, marinate the tofu and vegetables in the olive oil mixture for about 15 minutes before grilling.

# Caprese Baguette with Pesto Mayo

Serving: 4 | Prep Time: 10 minutes | Cook Time: 10 minutes

Ingredients:

- 12 oz (340 g) French baguette, cut into four equal sections
- 4 oz (113 g) fresh mozzarella cheese, thinly sliced
- 2 large tomatoes, thinly sliced
- 2 oz (57 g) fresh basil leaves
- 2 oz (57 g) sun-dried tomatoes (dry-packed), sliced
- 4 tbsp mayonnaise
- 2 tbsp pesto sauce
- 1 tbsp balsamic vinegar
- 1 tsp olive oil
- Salt and black pepper to taste

Directions:

1. Preheat your oven to 350°F (175°C).
2. In a small bowl, mix the mayonnaise and pesto sauce to create the pesto mayo.
3. Cut the baguette sections in half lengthwise, creating a top and bottom piece for each.
4. Place the baguette halves on a baking sheet and lightly toast them in the oven for about 5 minutes, or until they are slightly crisp.
5. Remove the toasted baguette from the oven and let it cool for a minute.
6. Spread the pesto mayo on both the top and bottom halves of each baguette section.
7. Layer fresh mozzarella slices, tomato slices, and sun-dried tomato pieces on the bottom half.
8. Sprinkle with fresh basil leaves, drizzle with balsamic vinegar and olive oil, and season with salt and black pepper.
9. Place the top halves of the baguette over the ingredients to create sandwiches.
10. Serve your Caprese Baguette with Pesto Mayo immediately.

Nutritional Values: Calories: 450 kcal | Fat: 21 g | Protein: 13 g | Carbs: 51 g | Net Carbs: 42 g | Fiber: 9 g | Cholesterol: 30 mg | Sodium: 500 mg | Potassium: 520 mg

Useful Tip: For an extra layer of flavor, you can add a balsamic reduction over the tomato and mozzarella layers.

# FISH AND SEAFOOD RECIPES

## Lemon-Herb Baked Salmon with Asparagus

Serving: 4 | Prep Time: 10 minutes | Cook Time: 20 minutes

**Ingredients:**

- 4 salmon fillets, 5 oz (140 g) each
- 1 lb (450 g) asparagus, woody ends trimmed
- 2 tbsp olive oil
- 2 cloves garlic, minced
- Zest of 1 lemon
- Juice of 1 lemon
- 2 tsp fresh thyme leaves
- Salt and black pepper, to taste
- Lemon slices for garnish

**Directions:**

1. Preheat your oven to 375°F (190°C).
2. Place the salmon fillets on a baking sheet lined with parchment paper.
3. In a bowl, mix the olive oil, minced garlic, lemon zest, lemon juice, and fresh thyme leaves.
4. Drizzle this mixture evenly over the salmon fillets.
5. Season the salmon with salt and black pepper.
6. Arrange the trimmed asparagus around the salmon fillets on the baking sheet.
7. Drizzle a little olive oil over the asparagus and season with salt and pepper.
8. Place lemon slices on top of the salmon fillets.
9. Bake in the preheated oven for 15-20 minutes or until the salmon flakes easily with a fork and the asparagus is tender.
10. Remove from the oven, garnish with additional fresh thyme if desired, and serve your Lemon-Herb Baked Salmon with Asparagus.

**Nutritional Values:** Calories: 340 kcal | Fat: 20 g | Protein: 30 g | Carbs: 10 g | Net Carbs: 5 g | Fiber: 5 g | Cholesterol: 75 mg | Sodium: 180 mg | Potassium: 900 mg

**Useful Tip:** For added flavor, you can marinate the salmon in the olive oil, garlic, lemon zest, lemon juice, and thyme mixture for 30 minutes before baking.

## Garlic Butter Shrimp Scampi

Serving: 4 | Prep Time: 10 minutes | Cook Time: 10 minutes

**Ingredients:**

- 1 lb (450 g) large shrimp, peeled and deveined
- 4 tbsp unsalted butter
- 4 cloves garlic, minced
- 1/4 tsp red pepper flakes (optional)
- Salt and black pepper, to taste
- Juice of 1 lemon
- Fresh parsley, chopped, for garnish
- Grated Parmesan cheese, for serving

## Directions:

1. In a large skillet, melt the butter over medium heat.
2. Add the minced garlic and red pepper flakes (if using) to the skillet, sautéing until the garlic becomes fragrant.
3. Add the shrimp to the skillet and cook until they turn pink, about 2-3 minutes per side. Season with salt and black pepper to taste.
4. Squeeze the juice of one lemon over the shrimp and stir to combine.
5. Remove from heat and garnish with chopped fresh parsley.
6. Serve hot, topped with grated Parmesan cheese.

**Nutritional Values:** Calories: 300 kcal | Fat: 18 g | Protein: 26 g | Carbs: 4 g | Net Carbs: 2 g | Fiber: 2 g | Cholesterol: 230 mg | Sodium: 300 mg | Potassium: 350 mg

**Useful Tip:** You can serve this delicious garlic butter shrimp scampi over a bed of fresh spinach or arugula for a low-carb, keto-friendly option.

# Blackened Catfish with Quinoa Pilaf

Serving: 4 | Prep Time: 15 minutes | Cook Time: 20 minutes

## Ingredients:

- 4 catfish fillets (16 oz / 450 g)
- 2 tbsp unsalted butter
- 2 tsp paprika
- 1 tsp dried thyme
- 1 tsp garlic powder
- 1/2 tsp onion powder
- 1/2 tsp cayenne pepper (adjust to taste)
- Salt and black pepper, to taste
- 6 oz (185 g) quinoa, rinsed
- 16 oz (475 ml) chicken or vegetable broth
- 2 oz (75 g) red bell pepper, diced
- 2 oz (75 g) yellow bell pepper, diced
- 2 oz (75 g) zucchini, diced
- 1 oz (30 g) red onion, finely chopped
- 2 oz (60 ml) fresh lemon juice
- Fresh parsley, chopped, for garnish
- Lemon wedges, for serving

## Directions:

1. In a small bowl, combine the paprika, dried thyme, garlic powder, onion powder, cayenne pepper, salt, and black pepper. This is your blackening seasoning.
2. Rub the blackening seasoning evenly over both sides of each catfish fillet.
3. In a large skillet, melt the butter over medium-high heat.
4. Add the catfish fillets to the skillet and cook for about 3-4 minutes on each side, or until the fish flakes easily with a fork. Remove from the skillet and keep warm.
5. In a separate saucepan, bring the chicken or vegetable broth to a boil.
6. Add the rinsed quinoa to the boiling broth, reduce heat to a simmer, and cook for about 15 minutes or until the quinoa is tender and the liquid is absorbed.
7. While the quinoa cooks, prepare the quinoa pilaf. In a large bowl, combine the cooked quinoa, diced red and yellow bell peppers, zucchini, and red onion.
8. Drizzle fresh lemon juice over the pilaf and toss to combine.
9. Serve the blackened catfish fillets on a bed of quinoa pilaf, garnished with chopped fresh parsley and lemon wedges.

Nutritional Values: Calories: 400 kcal | Fat: 12 g | Protein: 30 g | Carbs: 45 g | Net Carbs: 40 g | Fiber: 5 g | Cholesterol: 80 mg | Sodium: 600 mg | Potassium: 800 mg

Useful Tip: Adjust the amount of cayenne pepper in the blackening seasoning to control the spiciness of the dish.

## Cajun Spiced Tilapia Tacos

Serving: 4 | Prep Time: 15 minutes | Cook Time: 10 minutes

Ingredients:

- 16 oz (450 g) tilapia fillets
- 2 tbsp Cajun seasoning
- 2 tbsp olive oil
- 8 oz (240 ml) Greek yogurt
- 2 tbsp fresh lime juice
- 4 oz (150 g) red cabbage, shredded
- 2 oz (75 g) red onion, finely chopped
- 2 oz (75 g) red bell pepper, diced
- 2 oz (75 g) yellow bell pepper, diced
- 1 oz (60 ml) fresh cilantro, chopped
- 1 tsp garlic powder
- Salt and black pepper, to taste
- 8 small whole wheat tortillas
- Lime wedges, for serving

Directions:

1. In a small bowl, combine the Cajun seasoning, salt, and black pepper. This is your Cajun spice rub.
2. Rub the Cajun spice rub evenly over both sides of each tilapia fillet.
3. In a large skillet, heat the olive oil over medium-high heat.
4. Add the tilapia fillets to the skillet and cook for about 2-3 minutes per side or until the fish flakes easily with a fork. Remove from the skillet and keep warm.
5. In a medium bowl, prepare the lime-cilantro yogurt sauce by combining the Greek yogurt, fresh lime juice, garlic powder, and fresh cilantro. Mix well.
6. To assemble the tacos, warm the whole wheat tortillas according to the package instructions.
7. Place a portion of Cajun-spiced tilapia on each tortilla.
8. Top with shredded red cabbage, chopped red onion, red and yellow bell peppers, and a generous drizzle of lime-cilantro yogurt sauce.
9. Serve the tacos with lime wedges on the side.

Nutritional Values: Calories: 320 kcal | Fat: 8 g | Protein: 25 g | Carbs: 35 g | Net Carbs: 30 g | Fiber: 5 g | Cholesterol: 60 mg | Sodium: 400 mg | Potassium: 650 mg

Useful Tip: You can adjust the level of spiciness by adding more or less Cajun seasoning to the tilapia.

## Grilled Swordfish Steaks with Mango Salsa

Serving: 4 | Prep Time: 15 minutes | Cook Time: 10 minutes

Ingredients:

- 4 swordfish steaks, 6 oz (170 g) each
- 2 tbsp olive oil
- 1 tsp paprika
- 1 tsp cayenne pepper
- Salt and black pepper, to taste

For the Mango Salsa:

- 2 ripe mangoes, peeled, pitted, and diced
- 1/2 red onion, finely chopped
- 1 red bell pepper, diced
- 0,5 oz (15 g) fresh cilantro, chopped
- 1 jalapeño pepper, seeded and minced
- 2 tbsp fresh lime juice
- Salt and black pepper, to taste

**Directions:**

1. Preheat your grill to medium-high heat, about 400°F (200°C).
2. In a small bowl, combine the olive oil, paprika, cayenne pepper, salt, and black pepper. This is your spice rub for the swordfish.
3. Brush the spice rub over both sides of the swordfish steaks.
4. In a separate bowl, combine all the mango salsa ingredients: diced mangoes, finely chopped red onion, diced red bell pepper, minced jalapeño, fresh cilantro, and fresh lime juice. Add salt and black pepper to taste.
5. Grill the swordfish steaks for about 3-4 minutes per side or until they are no longer translucent and flake easily with a fork.
6. Remove the grilled swordfish from the grill and let them rest for a few minutes.
7. Serve the swordfish steaks topped with the fresh mango salsa.

**Nutritional Values:** Calories: 320 kcal | Fat: 10 g | Protein: 35 g | Carbs: 25 g | Net Carbs: 20 g | Fiber: 5 g | Cholesterol: 75 mg | Sodium: 300 mg | Potassium: 950 mg

**Useful Tip:** You can control the level of spiciness by adjusting the amount of cayenne pepper and jalapeño in the salsa.

## Mediterranean-Style Baked Cod

Serving: 4 | Prep Time: 15 minutes | Cook Time: 20 minutes

**Ingredients:**

- 4 cod fillets, 6 oz (170 g) each
- 2 tbsp olive oil
- 1 lemon, zested and juiced
- 3 cloves garlic, minced
- 1 tsp dried oregano
- 1 tsp dried basil
- 2 oz (75 g) Kalamata olives, pitted and chopped
- 1 oz (30 g) sun-dried tomatoes, chopped
- 1 oz (40 g) feta cheese, crumbled
- Salt and black pepper, to taste
- Fresh parsley, chopped, for garnish

**Directions:**

1. Preheat your oven to 375°F (190°C). Grease a baking dish with olive oil.
2. Place the cod fillets in the prepared baking dish.
3. In a small bowl, whisk together the olive oil, lemon zest, lemon juice, minced garlic, dried oregano, and dried basil. Pour this mixture over the cod fillets.
4. Sprinkle the chopped Kalamata olives and sun-dried tomatoes over the cod fillets.
5. Season with salt and black pepper to taste.
6. Cover the baking dish with foil and bake in the preheated oven for about 15 minutes.
7. Remove the foil and bake for an additional 5 minutes or until the cod flakes easily with a fork.
8. Sprinkle the crumbled feta cheese over the cod, and garnish with fresh chopped parsley.
9. Serve the Mediterranean-style baked cod with your choice of sides.

**Nutritional Values:** Calories: 290 kcal | Fat: 14 g | Protein: 32 g | Carbs: 11 g | Net Carbs: 8 g | Fiber: 3 g | Cholesterol: 70 mg | Sodium: 620 mg | Potassium: 900 mg

**Useful Tip:** You can add a drizzle of extra-virgin olive oil and a squeeze of fresh lemon juice for extra flavor just before serving.

## Thai-Style Coconut Curry Shrimp

Serving: 4 | Prep Time: 15 minutes | Cook Time: 20 minutes

**Ingredients:**

- 1 lb (450 g) large shrimp, peeled and deveined
- 1 can (13.5 oz or 400 ml) coconut milk
- 2 tbsp red curry paste
- 1 red bell pepper, sliced
- 1 yellow bell pepper, sliced
- 1 zucchini, sliced
- 1 onion, thinly sliced
- 2 cloves garlic, minced
- 1-inch (2.5 cm) piece of fresh ginger, grated
- 1 tbsp fish sauce
- 1 tsp brown sugar
- Juice of 1 lime
- Fresh cilantro leaves, for garnish
- Salt and pepper, to taste
- 2 tbsp vegetable oil

**Directions:**

1. Heat the vegetable oil in a large skillet over medium-high heat.
2. Add the sliced onion and cook until translucent.
3. Stir in the minced garlic and grated ginger, and cook for another minute.
4. Add the red curry paste to the skillet and cook for 2-3 minutes, stirring constantly to release the flavors.
5. Pour in the coconut milk and stir until the curry paste is well incorporated.
6. Add the sliced bell peppers and zucchini to the skillet. Simmer for 5-7 minutes or until the vegetables are tender.
7. Season with fish sauce, brown sugar, lime juice, salt, and pepper.
8. Gently stir in the shrimp and cook until they turn pink and opaque, about 3-4 minutes.
9. Remove the skillet from heat.
10. Garnish with fresh cilantro leaves.
11. Serve the Thai-style coconut curry shrimp over steamed jasmine rice or with your choice of side.

**Nutritional Values:** Calories: 320 kcal | Fat: 22 g | Protein: 18 g | Carbs: 18 g | Net Carbs: 12 g | Fiber: 6 g | Cholesterol: 120 mg | Sodium: 650 mg | Potassium: 550 mg

**Useful Tip:** For a spicier curry, increase the amount of red curry paste, or for a milder version, use less.

## Teriyaki Glazed Salmon with Sesame Broccoli

Serving: 4 | Prep Time: 15 minutes | Cook Time: 20 minutes

**Ingredients:**

- 4 salmon fillets, 6 oz (170 g) each
- 1 lb (450 g) broccoli florets
- 2 oz (60 ml) low-sodium soy sauce
- 2 tbsp mirin (rice wine)
- 2 tbsp honey
- 1 tsp fresh ginger, minced

- 1 tsp fresh garlic, minced
- 1 tbsp sesame oil
- 2 tbsp sesame seeds
- Salt and pepper, to taste
- Sliced green onions, for garnish
- Cooked white rice, for serving

**Directions:**

1. In a bowl, whisk together soy sauce, mirin, honey, minced ginger, and minced garlic to create the teriyaki glaze.
2. Season salmon fillets with salt and pepper. Place them in a zip-top bag or shallow dish, and pour half of the teriyaki glaze over them. Seal the bag or cover the dish and marinate for 15 minutes.
3. Preheat your grill or grill pan over medium-high heat.
4. While the grill is heating, steam the broccoli florets until tender, about 4-5 minutes.
5. Drizzle sesame oil over the steamed broccoli and sprinkle sesame seeds on top.
6. Grill the salmon fillets for about 4-5 minutes per side, brushing with the remaining teriyaki glaze while grilling.
7. While grilling, cook the remaining teriyaki glaze in a small saucepan until it thickens slightly, then set it aside.
8. Serve the teriyaki glazed salmon over cooked white rice with sesame broccoli on the side.
9. Drizzle the reserved teriyaki glaze over the salmon and garnish with sliced green onions.

**Nutritional Values:** Calories: 350 kcal | Fat: 12 g | Protein: 30 g | Carbs: 30 g | Net Carbs: 26 g | Fiber: 4 g | Cholesterol: 75 mg | Sodium: 720 mg | Potassium: 850 mg

**Useful Tip:** You can also broil the salmon in the oven for 10-12 minutes if you don't have a grill.

## Herb-Crusted Baked Halibut

Serving: 4 | Prep Time: 15 minutes | Cook Time: 20 minutes

**Ingredients:**

- 4 halibut fillets, 6 oz (170 g) each
- 3.5 oz (100 g) fresh breadcrumbs
- 0.88 oz (25 g) grated Parmesan cheese
- 2 oz (60 ml) olive oil
- 2 cloves garlic, minced
- 2 tbsp fresh lemon juice
- 1 tbsp Dijon mustard
- 0.5 oz (15 g) fresh parsley, chopped
- 0.5 oz (15 g) fresh basil, chopped
- Salt and pepper, to taste
- Lemon wedges, for garnish

**Directions:**

1. Preheat your oven to 375°F (190°C) and line a baking sheet with parchment paper.
2. In a bowl, combine fresh breadcrumbs, grated Parmesan cheese, minced garlic, chopped parsley, chopped basil, and a pinch of salt and pepper.
3. In a separate bowl, whisk together olive oil, fresh lemon juice, and Dijon mustard.
4. Brush each halibut fillet with the olive oil mixture.
5. Press the breadcrumb mixture onto the tops of the halibut fillets, creating a generous crust.
6. Place the herb-crusted halibut fillets on the prepared baking sheet.
7. Bake in the preheated oven for 15-20 minutes or until the fish flakes easily with a fork and the crust is golden brown.
8. Garnish with lemon wedges and serve.

Nutritional Values: Calories: 370 kcal | Fat: 20 g | Protein: 35 g | Carbs: 11 g | Net Carbs: 7 g | Fiber: 4 g | Cholesterol: 75 mg | Sodium: 350 mg | Potassium: 750 mg

Useful Tip: You can customize the herb crust with your favorite fresh herbs and adjust the seasoning to your preference.

# Pesto Grilled Shrimp Skewers

Serving: 4 | Prep Time: 15 minutes | Cook Time: 6 minutes

Ingredients:

- 16 large shrimp, peeled and deveined, about 12 oz (340 g)
- 2.4 oz (60 ml) pesto sauce
- 2 cloves garlic, minced
- 2 tbsp olive oil
- 1 tbsp lemon juice
- 1 tsp balsamic vinegar
- 1 tsp red pepper flakes (adjust to taste)
- Salt and pepper, to taste
- 4 metal or wooden skewers, soaked in water (if using wooden skewers)
- Fresh basil leaves, for garnish

Directions:

1. Preheat your grill to medium-high heat, around 400°F (200°C).
2. In a bowl, combine pesto sauce, minced garlic, olive oil, lemon juice, balsamic vinegar, red pepper flakes, salt, and pepper.
3. Thread four shrimp onto each skewer, making sure to pierce through both the tail and the head of each shrimp.
4. Brush the shrimp skewers generously with the pesto mixture, coating them evenly.
5. Place the shrimp skewers on the preheated grill and cook for about 2-3 minutes per side, or until they turn pink and slightly charred.
6. Once cooked, remove the shrimp skewers from the grill and drizzle any remaining pesto mixture over them.
7. Garnish with fresh basil leaves.
8. Serve your Pesto Grilled Shrimp Skewers with your choice of side dishes.

Nutritional Values: Calories: 240 kcal | Fat: 18 g | Protein: 18 g | Carbs: 2 g | Net Carbs: 1 g | Fiber: 1 g | Cholesterol: 150 mg | Sodium: 370 mg | Potassium: 190 mg

Useful Tip: Soak wooden skewers in water for about 30 minutes before using them to prevent burning on the grill.

# Harissa Spiced Sea Bass with Couscous

Serving: 4 | Prep Time: 15 minutes | Cook Time: 15 minutes

Ingredients:

- 4 sea bass fillets, about 5 oz (140 g) each
- 2 tbsp olive oil
- 2 tbsp harissa paste
- 7 oz (200 g) couscous
- 12.2 oz (360 ml) vegetable broth
- 2.6 oz (75 g) diced bell peppers (red, yellow, or green)
- 1.1 oz (30 g) diced red onion
- 1.2 oz (35 g) diced zucchini
- 1.2 oz (35 g) diced tomatoes
- 1.1 oz (30 g) diced cucumber

- 1.2 oz (35 g) chopped fresh cilantro
- 1 fl oz (30 ml) fresh lemon juice
- 0.2 oz (5 g) ground cumin
- Salt and pepper, to taste
- Lemon wedges, for garnish

## Directions:

1. Preheat your grill to medium-high heat, about 200°C (400°F).
2. In a small bowl, mix the olive oil and harissa paste. Brush this mixture evenly onto the sea bass fillets and let them marinate for 10 minutes.
3. While the sea bass is marinating, prepare the couscous. In a saucepan, bring the vegetable broth to a boil, then pour it over the couscous in a heatproof bowl. Cover the bowl with a lid or plastic wrap and let it sit for 5 minutes. Fluff the couscous with a fork and set it aside.
4. Grill the sea bass fillets for about 3-4 minutes per side or until they are cooked through and have grill marks.
5. In a large mixing bowl, combine the diced bell peppers, red onion, zucchini, tomatoes, cucumber, cilantro, lemon juice, and cumin. Toss the ingredients to mix them well.
6. Add the prepared couscous to the vegetable mixture and gently combine them.
7. Season the couscous salad with salt and pepper to taste.
8. Serve the grilled harissa-spiced sea bass fillets on a bed of couscous salad, garnished with lemon wedges.

**Nutritional Values:** Calories: 380 kcal | Fat: 11 g | Protein: 28 g | Carbs: 40 g | Net Carbs: 33 g | Fiber: 7 g | Cholesterol: 55 mg | Sodium: 450 mg | Potassium: 580 mg

**Useful Tip:** When grilling fish, it's essential not to overcook it. Sea bass is ready when it flakes easily with a fork.

# Chimichurri Marinated Grilled Tuna

Serving: 4 | Prep Time: 15 minutes | Cook Time: 8-10 minutes

## Ingredients:

- 4 tuna steaks, 6 oz (170 g) each
- 0.5 oz (15 g) fresh parsley leaves
- 0.3 oz (10 g) fresh cilantro leaves
- 0.2 oz (5 g) fresh oregano leaves
- 4 cloves garlic
- 1.4 oz (40 ml) red wine vinegar
- 3.5 oz (100 ml) olive oil
- 0.1 oz (3 g) red pepper flakes
- Salt and pepper, to taste
- 1 lemon, cut into wedges

## Directions:

1. In a food processor, combine the fresh parsley, cilantro, oregano, garlic, red wine vinegar, and red pepper flakes. Pulse until finely chopped.
2. With the food processor running, slowly drizzle in the olive oil until the mixture forms a smooth sauce. Season with salt and pepper to taste.
3. Place the tuna steaks in a shallow dish and coat them with half of the chimichurri sauce. Reserve the other half for serving.
4. Let the tuna marinate for at least 15 minutes at room temperature or longer in the refrigerator.
5. Preheat your grill to high heat, about 230°C (450°F).
6. Grill the marinated tuna steaks for 2-3 minutes per side, depending on your desired doneness. Tuna is typically served rare to medium-rare.
7. Remove the tuna steaks from the grill and let them rest for a few minutes.

8. Serve the grilled tuna steaks drizzled with the reserved chimichurri sauce and lemon wedges on the side.

**Nutritional Values:** Calories: 300 kcal | Fat: 18 g | Protein: 32 g | Carbs: 3 g | Net Carbs: 2 g | Fiber: 1 g | Cholesterol: 45 mg | Sodium: 220 mg | Potassium: 450 mg

**Useful Tip:** To keep the tuna moist and flavorful, avoid overcooking. Tuna should be seared on the outside and still pink in the center.

## Lemon-Dill Baked Trout with Steamed Greens

Serving: 4 | Prep Time: 15 minutes | Cook Time: 20 minutes

**Ingredients:**

- 4 trout fillets, 6 oz (170 g) each
- 1 lemon, thinly sliced
- 1.4 oz (40 ml) olive oil
- 1 oz (30 g) fresh dill, chopped
- 2 cloves garlic, minced
- Salt and pepper, to taste
- 1 lb (450 g) mixed greens (spinach, kale, or Swiss chard)
- 1.4 oz (40 ml) water
- Lemon wedges, for serving

**Directions:**

1. Preheat your oven to 200°C (400°F).
2. In a small bowl, combine the olive oil, fresh dill, minced garlic, salt, and pepper.
3. Lay out four large pieces of aluminum foil, one for each trout fillet. Place a handful of mixed greens in the center of each foil piece.
4. Season the trout fillets with salt and pepper, then place one fillet on top of the bed of greens on each piece of foil.
5. Drizzle the olive oil and dill mixture over the trout fillets.
6. Lay lemon slices over each fillet, and then fold up the sides of the foil to create packets, sealing them tightly.
7. Place the foil packets on a baking sheet and bake for 15-20 minutes or until the trout flakes easily with a fork.
8. While the trout is baking, steam the remaining mixed greens with 1.4 oz (40 ml) of water in a covered pot for 3-5 minutes or until wilted.
9. Serve the baked trout over the steamed greens, drizzling any juices from the foil packets over the top. Garnish with lemon wedges.

**Nutritional Values:** Calories: 280 kcal | Fat: 15 g | Protein: 32 g | Carbs: 7 g | Net Carbs: 3 g | Fiber: 4 g | Cholesterol: 85 mg | Sodium: 90 mg | Potassium: 650 mg

**Useful Tip:** Cooking fish in foil packets helps seal in moisture and flavor, resulting in tender, juicy fish.

## Miso-Glazed Cod with Roasted Brussels Sprouts

Serving: 4 | Prep Time: 15 minutes | Cook Time: 20 minutes

**Ingredients:**

- 4 cod fillets, 6 oz (170 g) each
- 1 lb (450 g) Brussels sprouts, trimmed and halved
- 1.4 oz (40 ml) olive oil
- 3 tablespoons (45 ml) white miso paste
- 1.4 oz (40 ml) rice vinegar

- 1.4 oz (40 ml) honey
- 2 cloves garlic, minced
- Salt and pepper, to taste
- Chopped fresh parsley for garnish

**Directions:**

1. Preheat your oven to 200°C (400°F).
2. In a large bowl, toss the halved Brussels sprouts with 1.4 oz (40 ml) of olive oil, salt, and pepper. Spread them out on a baking sheet.
3. Roast the Brussels sprouts in the preheated oven for 20 minutes or until they are tender and lightly browned.
4. While the Brussels sprouts are roasting, in a small bowl, whisk together the white miso paste, rice vinegar, honey, and minced garlic.
5. Season the cod fillets with salt and pepper and brush the miso glaze evenly over the fillets.
6. Remove the Brussels sprouts from the oven and make space on the baking sheet for the cod fillets.
7. Place the glazed cod fillets on the baking sheet alongside the Brussels sprouts.
8. Return the baking sheet to the oven and bake for an additional 10 minutes or until the cod is cooked through and flakes easily with a fork.
9. Garnish with chopped fresh parsley before serving.

**Nutritional Values:** Calories: 290 kcal | Fat: 10 g | Protein: 30 g | Carbs: 20 g | Net Carbs: 12 g | Fiber: 8 g | Cholesterol: 60 mg | Sodium: 650 mg | Potassium: 800 mg

**Useful Tip:** For a touch of freshness, you can also squeeze some lemon juice over the cod and Brussels sprouts just before serving.

## Mediterranean Zucchini and Shrimp Stir-Fry

Serving: 4 | Prep Time: 15 minutes | Cook Time: 15 minutes

**Ingredients:**

- 16 oz (450 g) large shrimp, peeled and deveined
- 16 oz (450 g) zucchinis, spiralized or cut into thin strips
- 1 red bell pepper, thinly sliced
- 2 oz (60 ml) olive oil
- 4 cloves garlic, minced
- 1 tsp dried oregano
- 1/2 tsp dried basil
- Salt and pepper, to taste
- Juice of 1 lemon
- Crumbled feta cheese for garnish
- Fresh basil leaves for garnish

**Directions:**

1. In a large skillet or wok, heat the olive oil over medium-high heat.
2. Add the minced garlic and sauté for about 1 minute until fragrant.
3. Add the sliced red bell pepper and sauté for another 2 minutes until it begins to soften.
4. Add the shrimp to the skillet and stir-fry for 2-3 minutes until they turn pink and opaque. Remove the cooked shrimp and bell peppers from the skillet and set them aside.
5. In the same skillet, add the spiralized or thinly sliced zucchinis, dried oregano, dried basil, salt, and pepper (to taste).
6. Stir-fry the zucchinis for about 3-4 minutes until they are tender yet still crisp.
7. Return the cooked shrimp and red bell peppers to the skillet and stir to combine with the zucchinis.

8. Squeeze the juice of one lemon over the stir-fry and give it one final stir.

9. Serve the Mediterranean zucchini and shrimp stir-fry garnished with crumbled feta cheese and fresh basil leaves.

**Nutritional Values:** Calories: 260 kcal | Fat: 15 g | Protein: 25 g | Carbs: 10 g | Net Carbs: 7 g | Fiber: 3 g | Cholesterol: 180 mg | Sodium: 350 mg | Potassium: 600 mg

**Useful Tip:** Don't overcook the zucchinis; they should maintain a slightly crisp texture for the perfect stir-fry.

## Turmeric and Coconut Mussels

Serving: 4 | Prep Time: 10 minutes | Cook Time: 15 minutes

**Ingredients:**

- 32 oz (900 g) fresh mussels, cleaned and debearded
- 13.5 oz (400 ml) coconut milk
- 1 onion, finely chopped
- 2 cloves garlic, minced
- 1 tbsp olive oil
- 1 tsp ground turmeric
- 1/2 tsp red pepper flakes (adjust to taste)
- Salt and black pepper, to taste
- Fresh cilantro leaves for garnish
- 1 lime, cut into wedges

**Directions:**

1. In a large saucepan, heat the olive oil over medium heat.
2. Add the finely chopped onion and sauté for about 3 minutes until it turns translucent.
3. Stir in the minced garlic, ground turmeric, and red pepper flakes; cook for an additional minute to release their flavors.
4. Add the cleaned mussels to the saucepan and pour in the coconut milk.
5. Cover the saucepan with a lid and simmer for about 5-7 minutes, or until the mussels have opened (discard any that remain closed).
6. Season the mussels with salt and black pepper to taste.
7. Ladle the mussels and the aromatic broth into serving bowls.
8. Garnish with fresh cilantro leaves and serve with lime wedges.

**Nutritional Values:** Calories: 300 kcal | Fat: 20 g | Protein: 12 g | Carbs: 10 g | Net Carbs: 5 g | Fiber: 5 g | Cholesterol: 30 mg | Sodium: 500 mg | Potassium: 600 mg

**Useful Tip:** Ensure that the mussels are cleaned and debearded before cooking to remove any sand or debris, and discard any mussels that do not open after cooking.

## Lemon-Thyme Roasted Red Snapper

Serving: 4 | Prep Time: 10 minutes | Cook Time: 20 minutes

**Ingredients:**

- 4 red snapper fillets, about 6 oz (170 g) each
- 2 tbsp olive oil
- 2 lemons, zested and juiced
- 2 tbsp fresh thyme leaves
- 2 cloves garlic, minced
- Salt and black pepper, to taste

- Lemon slices and fresh thyme sprigs for garnish

## Directions:

1. Preheat your oven to 400°F (200°C).
2. In a small bowl, combine the olive oil, lemon zest, lemon juice, fresh thyme leaves, and minced garlic.
3. Place the red snapper fillets on a baking sheet lined with parchment paper.
4. Brush the fillets with the lemon-thyme mixture, ensuring they are evenly coated.
5. Season the fillets with salt and black pepper to taste.
6. Roast the red snapper in the preheated oven for about 15-20 minutes, or until the fish is cooked through and flakes easily with a fork.
7. Garnish with lemon slices and fresh thyme sprigs.

**Nutritional Values:** Calories: 280 kcal | Fat: 12 g | Protein: 40 g | Carbs: 6 g | Net Carbs: 4 g | Fiber: 2 g | Cholesterol: 60 mg | Sodium: 300 mg | Potassium: 550 mg

**Useful Tip:** Adjust the roasting time based on the thickness of your red snapper fillets. Thicker fillets may require a few extra minutes in the oven.

## Balsamic-Glazed Scallops with Spinach

Serving: 4 | Prep Time: 15 minutes | Cook Time: 10 minutes

## Ingredients:

- 16 large sea scallops, about 20 oz (560 g)
- 2 tbsp olive oil
- 2 cloves garlic, minced
- 2.5 oz (75 ml) balsamic vinegar
- 2.5 oz (75 ml) chicken broth
- 2 tbsp honey
- 4 oz (120 g) fresh spinach
- Salt and black pepper, to taste
- Fresh basil leaves for garnish

## Directions:

1. Pat the scallops dry with a paper towel and season them with salt and black pepper.
2. In a large skillet, heat the olive oil over medium-high heat.
3. Add the scallops to the skillet and sear for about 2-3 minutes on each side until they are browned and cooked through. Remove the scallops from the skillet and set them aside.
4. In the same skillet, add the minced garlic and sauté for about 1 minute until fragrant.
5. Stir in the balsamic vinegar, chicken broth, and honey. Allow the mixture to simmer and reduce until it thickens, which should take about 5 minutes.
6. Return the scallops to the skillet and coat them with the balsamic glaze.
7. Add the fresh spinach to the skillet and cook for 2-3 minutes, or until it wilts.
8. Garnish with fresh basil leaves.

**Nutritional Values:** Calories: 280 kcal | Fat: 8 g | Protein: 30 g | Carbs: 14 g | Net Carbs: 12 g | Fiber: 2 g | Cholesterol: 60 mg | Sodium: 350 mg | Potassium: 550 mg

**Useful Tip:** Be careful not to overcook the scallops, as they can become tough. They should be opaque and slightly firm to the touch.

# Mediterranean-Style Stuffed Squid

Serving: 4 | Prep Time: 20 minutes | Cook Time: 35 minutes

Ingredients:

- 8 medium-sized squid tubes (about 24 oz or 680 g)
- 8 oz (240 ml) cooked quinoa
- 8 oz (225 g) diced tomatoes
- 4 oz (115 g) feta cheese, crumbled
- 2 cloves garlic, minced
- 2 oz (60 ml) fresh lemon juice
- 2 oz (60 ml) extra-virgin olive oil
- 2 oz (60 ml) chopped fresh parsley
- 2 oz (60 ml) chopped fresh mint
- 2 oz (60 ml) chopped fresh basil
- Salt and black pepper, to taste
- Lemon wedges, for serving

Directions:

1. Preheat your oven to 350°F (175°C).
2. In a large mixing bowl, combine the cooked quinoa, diced tomatoes, feta cheese, minced garlic, fresh lemon juice, and extra-virgin olive oil.
3. Stir in the chopped fresh herbs: parsley, mint, and basil. Season with salt and black pepper to taste.
4. Gently stuff the squid tubes with the quinoa mixture, leaving some space at the top to allow for expansion.
5. Use toothpicks to secure the tops of the squid tubes.
6. Place the stuffed squid tubes in an oven-safe dish and drizzle with a bit of olive oil.
7. Cover the dish with foil and bake for 20-25 minutes, or until the squid is tender.
8. Remove the foil and broil for 5-10 minutes until the tops are golden brown.
9. Serve the Mediterranean-style stuffed squid with lemon wedges.

Nutritional Values: Calories: 300 kcal | Fat: 14 g | Protein: 22 g | Carbs: 24 g | Net Carbs: 21 g | Fiber: 3 g | Cholesterol: 100 mg | Sodium: 550 mg | Potassium: 580 mg

Useful Tip: Be careful not to overstuff the squid tubes as the quinoa will expand during cooking.

# Citrus-Marinated Grilled Mahi-Mahi

Serving: 4 | Prep Time: 15 minutes | Cook Time: 10 minutes

Ingredients:

- 4 Mahi-Mahi fillets, about 6 oz (170 g) each
- 2 oz (60 ml) fresh orange juice
- 2 oz (60 ml) fresh lime juice
- 2 tbsp fresh lemon juice
- 2 cloves garlic, minced
- 2 tbsp olive oil
- 1 tsp honey
- 1 tsp cumin
- 1 tsp paprika
- Salt and black pepper, to taste
- Fresh cilantro, for garnish
- Sliced citrus wedges, for serving

Directions:

1. In a bowl, whisk together the fresh orange juice, lime juice, lemon juice, minced garlic, olive oil, honey, cumin, paprika, salt, and black pepper.

2.  Place the Mahi-Mahi fillets in a resealable plastic bag or a shallow dish and pour the citrus marinade over them. Seal the bag or cover the dish, then refrigerate for at least 30 minutes, allowing the fish to marinate.
3.  Preheat your grill to medium-high heat (about 400°F or 200°C).
4.  Remove the Mahi-Mahi fillets from the marinade and let any excess drip off.
5.  Grill the fillets for about 4-5 minutes on each side, or until they easily flake with a fork and have beautiful grill marks.
6.  Garnish the grilled Mahi-Mahi with fresh cilantro and serve with sliced citrus wedges.

**Nutritional Values:** Calories: 250 kcal | Fat: 9 g | Protein: 35 g | Carbs: 6 g | Net Carbs: 5 g | Fiber: 1 g | Cholesterol: 140 mg | Sodium: 320 mg | Potassium: 780 mg

**Useful Tip:** When grilling fish, it's important not to overcook it. Fish is done when it flakes easily but is still moist in the center.

# POULTRY AND MEAT RECIPES

## Lemon-Rosemary Roasted Chicken

Serving: 4 | Prep Time: 15 minutes | Cook Time: 1 hour and 15 minutes

Ingredients:

- 1 whole chicken, about 4 lbs (1800 g)
- 2 oz (60 g) butter, softened
- 2 tbsp olive oil
- 1 lemon, zested and juiced
- 2 cloves garlic, minced
- 1 tbsp fresh rosemary, chopped
- Salt and black pepper, to taste
- 1 lemon, thinly sliced
- Fresh rosemary sprigs, for garnish

Directions:

1. Preheat your oven to 375°F (190°C).
2. In a bowl, combine the softened butter, olive oil, lemon zest, minced garlic, and chopped rosemary.
3. Season the chicken inside and out with salt and black pepper. Place a few lemon slices inside the chicken cavity.
4. Gently loosen the skin of the chicken without tearing it. Spread the rosemary butter mixture under the skin of the chicken, covering the breasts and thighs.
5. Squeeze the juice from the zested lemon over the chicken and place the remaining lemon slices on top.
6. Transfer the chicken to a roasting pan and add 1 cup (240 ml) of water to the pan.
7. Roast the chicken in the preheated oven for about 1 hour and 15 minutes or until the internal temperature reaches 165°F (74°C). Baste the chicken with the pan juices every 20-30 minutes.
8. Once done, remove the chicken from the oven and let it rest for 10 minutes before carving.
9. Garnish with fresh rosemary sprigs.

Nutritional Values: Calories: 420 kcal | Fat: 26 g | Protein: 40 g | Carbs: 4 g | Net Carbs: 2 g | Fiber: 2 g | Cholesterol: 140 mg | Sodium: 380 mg | Potassium: 450 mg

Useful Tip: For a more flavorful roast, let the chicken marinate with the rosemary butter mixture in the refrigerator for a few hours or overnight.

## Grilled Turkey Burgers with Avocado

Serving: 4 | Prep Time: 15 minutes | Cook Time: 12 minutes

Ingredients:

- 16 oz (450 g) ground turkey
- 2 oz (60 ml) low-sodium chicken broth
- 2.5 oz (70 g) breadcrumbs
- 2.5 oz (20 g) grated Parmesan cheese
- 1/2 small onion, finely chopped
- 1/2 tsp Worcestershire sauce
- 1/2 tsp garlic powder
- Salt and black pepper, to taste
- 4 whole-grain hamburger buns
- 1 ripe avocado, sliced

- Lettuce, tomato, and red onion slices for garnish

## Directions:

1. Preheat your grill to medium-high heat (about 375°F/190°C).
2. In a mixing bowl, combine the ground turkey, low-sodium chicken broth, chopped onion, breadcrumbs, grated Parmesan cheese, Worcestershire sauce, garlic powder, salt, and black pepper. Mix until well combined.
3. Divide the turkey mixture into 4 equal portions and shape them into burger patties.
4. Place the burger patties on the preheated grill. Grill for approximately 5-6 minutes per side, or until the internal temperature reaches 165°F (74°C).
5. During the last couple of minutes, toast the whole-grain buns on the grill until they are lightly browned.
6. To assemble the burgers, spread avocado slices on the bottom half of each bun. Place a turkey burger on top of the avocado, then add lettuce, tomato, and red onion slices. Top with the other half of the bun.
7. Serve your grilled turkey burgers with a side of your choice.

**Nutritional Values:** Calories: 330 kcal | Fat: 14 g | Protein: 29 g | Carbs: 25 g | Net Carbs: 20 g | Fiber: 5 g | Cholesterol: 75 mg | Sodium: 360 mg | Potassium: 500 mg

**Useful Tip:** Adding chicken broth to the turkey mixture helps keep the burgers moist and flavorful.

# Beef and Vegetable Stir-Fry

Serving: 4 | Prep Time: 15 minutes | Cook Time: 10 minutes

## Ingredients:

- 16 oz (450 g) lean beef strips
- 7 oz (200 g) broccoli florets
- 5 oz (140 g) snap peas
- 4 oz (115 g) carrots, thinly sliced
- 4 oz (115 g) bell peppers (assorted colors), sliced
- 4 oz (115 g) mushrooms, sliced
- 2 cloves garlic, minced
- 2 oz (60 ml) low-sodium soy sauce
- 2 oz (60 ml) beef broth
- 1 tbsp toasted sesame oil
- 2 tsp cornstarch
- 1 tsp honey
- 1/2 tsp ginger, minced
- 1/2 tsp crushed red pepper flakes (adjust to your desired spice level)
- 2 tbsp vegetable oil
- Sesame seeds for garnish
- Cooked brown rice for serving

## Directions:

1. In a small bowl, whisk together the low-sodium soy sauce, beef broth, toasted sesame oil, cornstarch, honey, minced ginger, and crushed red pepper flakes. Set aside.
2. Heat the vegetable oil in a large skillet or wok over high heat.
3. Add the beef strips and stir-fry for 2-3 minutes or until browned. Remove the beef from the skillet and set aside.
4. In the same skillet, add the minced garlic (2 cloves) and stir-fry for about 30 seconds, until fragrant.
5. Add the broccoli florets, snap peas, carrots, bell peppers, and mushrooms to the skillet. Stir-fry for 4-5 minutes until the vegetables are tender-crisp.

6. Return the cooked beef to the skillet and pour the sauce over the beef and vegetables. Stir-fry for an additional 2-3 minutes or until everything is well-coated and heated through.

7. Serve the stir-fry over cooked brown rice and garnish with sesame seeds.

**Nutritional Values:** Calories: 350 kcal | Fat: 12 g | Protein: 30 g | Carbs: 32 g | Net Carbs: 25 g | Fiber: 7 g | Cholesterol: 60 mg | Sodium: 750 mg | Potassium: 850 mg

**Useful Tip:** Feel free to customize this stir-fry with your favorite vegetables and adjust the level of spice according to your preference.

# Moroccan-Spiced Rabbit Stew

Serving: 4 | Prep time: 20 minutes | Cook time: 75 minutes

## Ingredients:

- 1.5 lb (680 g) rabbit meat, cut into pieces
- 2 tbsp olive oil
- 1 large onion, finely chopped
- 2 cloves garlic, minced
- 1 tsp ground cumin
- 1 tsp ground coriander
- 1 tsp ground paprika
- 1/2 tsp ground cinnamon
- 1/4 tsp cayenne pepper
- 14 oz (400 g) canned diced tomatoes
- 8 oz (240 ml) chicken broth
- 2 oz (75 g) pitted green olives
- 0,5 oz (15 g) chopped fresh cilantro
- Salt and pepper to taste

## Directions:

1. In a large pot, heat the olive oil over medium heat. Add the chopped onion and sauté until it becomes translucent, about 5 minutes.

2. Add the minced garlic and continue to sauté for another 1-2 minutes, until fragrant.

3. Stir in the ground cumin, coriander, paprika, cinnamon, and cayenne pepper. Cook for an additional 2 minutes, allowing the spices to bloom.

4. Add the rabbit pieces to the pot and brown them on all sides, about 5 minutes.

5. Pour in the diced tomatoes and chicken broth, then add the green olives. Bring the stew to a gentle boil.

6. Reduce the heat, cover the pot, and simmer for 1 hour, or until the rabbit meat becomes tender and easily shreds with a fork.

7. Season with salt and pepper to taste, then stir in the fresh cilantro. Simmer for an additional 10 minutes to allow the flavors to meld.

8. Serve the Moroccan-Spiced Rabbit Stew hot, garnished with extra cilantro if desired. Enjoy the dish.

**Nutritional Values:** Calories: 340 kcal | Fat: 15 g | Protein: 37 g | Carbs: 14 g | Net Carbs: 9 g | Fiber: 5 g | Cholesterol: 115 mg | Sodium: 970 mg | Potassium: 550 mg

**Useful Tip:** You can marinate the rabbit meat with the spices for a few hours or overnight for even more flavor.

# Teriyaki Pork Skewers

Serving: 4 | Prep time: 15 minutes | Cook time: 20 minutes

Ingredients:

- 20 oz (570 g) pork tenderloin, cut into 1-inch cubes
- 2 oz (60 ml) low-sodium soy sauce
- 2 tbsp honey
- 2 tbsp rice vinegar
- 1 tbsp mirin
- 1 tbsp sesame oil
- 2 cloves garlic, minced
- 1 tsp ginger, minced
- 1/4 tsp red pepper flakes
- 1 bell pepper, cut into 1-inch pieces
- 1 red onion, cut into 1-inch pieces
- Wooden skewers, soaked in water for 30 minutes

Directions:

1. In a bowl, whisk together the soy sauce, honey, rice vinegar, mirin, sesame oil, minced garlic, ginger, and red pepper flakes to make the teriyaki marinade.
2. Place the pork cubes in a resealable plastic bag or a shallow dish and pour half of the marinade over the pork. Seal the bag or cover the dish, and marinate in the refrigerator for at least 30 minutes.
3. Preheat your grill to medium-high heat (about 400°F/200°C).
4. Thread the marinated pork, bell pepper, and red onion alternately onto the soaked wooden skewers.
5. Grill the skewers for about 10 minutes, turning occasionally and basting with the reserved marinade until the pork is cooked through and slightly caramelized.
6. Serve the Teriyaki Pork Skewers hot and drizzle any remaining marinade over the top.

Nutritional Values: Calories: 280 kcal | Fat: 8 g | Protein: 30 g | Carbs: 20 g | Net carbs: 18 g | Fiber: 2 g | Cholesterol: 75 mg | Sodium: 550 mg | Potassium: 680 mg

Useful Tip: Marinate the pork for at least 30 minutes or overnight for more flavor.

# Quail in Red Wine Sauce

Serving: 4 | Prep time: 20 minutes | Cook time: 40 minutes

Ingredients:

- 4 quails (16 oz or 450 g each)
- 2 tbsp olive oil
- 2 shallots, finely chopped
- 2 cloves garlic, minced
- 8 oz (240 ml) dry red wine
- 4 oz (120 ml) chicken broth
- 2 sprigs fresh thyme
- 2 bay leaves
- Salt and pepper to taste
- 1 tbsp butter
- Fresh parsley for garnish

Directions:

1. Preheat your oven to 375°F (190°C).
2. Season the quails with salt and pepper, inside and out.
3. In a large ovenproof skillet, heat the olive oil over medium-high heat. Brown the quails on all sides until they're golden. Remove them from the skillet and set aside.

4. In the same skillet, add the chopped shallots and garlic. Sauté for a couple of minutes until they become fragrant and translucent.
5. Pour in the red wine and chicken broth, and add the thyme and bay leaves. Bring to a boil, then reduce to a simmer and let it cook for about 10 minutes or until the liquid reduces by half.
6. Return the quails to the skillet and transfer it to the preheated oven. Roast for 20-25 minutes, basting the quails with the sauce occasionally.
7. Remove the skillet from the oven, and stir in the butter to create a velvety red wine sauce.
8. Garnish with fresh parsley and serve your Quail in Red Wine Sauce hot.

**Nutritional Values:** Calories: 320 kcal | Fat: 12 g | Protein: 36 g | Carbs: 3 g | Net carbs: 2 g | Fiber: 1 g | Cholesterol: 105 mg | Sodium: 220 mg | Potassium: 520 mg

**Useful Tip:** To keep the quail tender, avoid overcooking; quail is done when the internal temperature reaches 160°F (71°C).

# Herbed Veal Medallions with Asparagus

Serving: 4 | Prep time: 15 minutes | Cook time: 20 minutes

## Ingredients:

- 16 oz (450 g) veal medallions
- 8 oz (225 g) asparagus spears, trimmed
- 2 tbsp olive oil
- 1 tsp garlic, minced
- 1 tsp fresh thyme, chopped
- 1 tsp fresh rosemary, chopped
- 1/2 tsp salt
- 1/4 tsp black pepper
- 4 oz (120 ml) white wine
- 4 oz (120 ml) chicken broth

## Directions:

1. Season the veal medallions with salt and pepper.
2. In a large skillet, heat the olive oil over medium-high heat and add the veal medallions. Sear for 2-3 minutes on each side until golden brown. Remove from the skillet and set aside.
3. In the same skillet, add the garlic, thyme, and rosemary. Sauté for 1 minute until fragrant.
4. Add the asparagus and sauté for 3-4 minutes until they become tender-crisp.
5. Pour in the white wine and chicken broth, and bring to a simmer. Cook for 2-3 minutes to reduce the liquid slightly.
6. Return the veal medallions to the skillet and cook for an additional 3-4 minutes until they are cooked to your desired level of doneness.
7. Serve the veal medallions on a plate with asparagus, spooning the herbed sauce over the top.

**Nutritional Values:** Calories: 320 kcal | Fat: 16 g | Protein: 34 g | Carbs: 6 g | Net carbs: 4 g | Fiber: 2 g | Cholesterol: 120 mg | Sodium: 580 mg | Potassium: 780 mg

**Useful Tip:** Pair this dish with a side of mashed potatoes or a simple green salad for a well-rounded meal.

# Garlic-Herb Grilled Chicken Thighs

Serving: 4 | Prep time: 10 minutes | Cook time: 15 minutes

Ingredients:

- 16 oz (450 g) boneless, skinless chicken thighs
- 2 tbsp olive oil
- 2 cloves garlic, minced
- 1 tsp dried oregano
- 1 tsp dried thyme
- 1/2 tsp salt
- 1/4 tsp black pepper
- 1 lemon, juiced
- 2 oz (60 ml) chicken broth

Directions:

1. In a bowl, combine the olive oil, minced garlic, dried oregano, dried thyme, salt, and black pepper.
2. Place the chicken thighs in a resealable plastic bag or shallow dish and pour the marinade over them. Seal the bag or cover the dish and refrigerate for at least 30 minutes, or marinate overnight for more flavor.
3. Preheat your grill to medium-high heat (about 375°F or 190°C).
4. Remove the chicken from the marinade and grill for 6-7 minutes per side, or until the internal temperature reaches 165°F (74°C) and the chicken is no longer pink in the center.
5. While grilling, baste the chicken with the lemon juice and chicken broth mixture for added flavor and moisture.
6. Once done, remove the chicken from the grill and let it rest for a few minutes before serving.
7. Serve with your favorite side dishes or a fresh salad.

Nutritional Values: Calories: 260 kcal | Fat: 14 g | Protein: 29 g | Carbs: 2 g | Net carbs: 1 g | Fiber: 1 g | Cholesterol: 120 mg | Sodium: 580 mg | Potassium: 380 mg

Useful Tip: For a delightful smoky flavor, add a few wood chips to the grill while cooking the chicken.

# Ground Beef and Mushroom Stuffed Bell Peppers

Serving: 4 | Prep time: 20 minutes | Cook time: 40 minutes

Ingredients:

- 4 bell peppers
- 16 oz (450 g) lean ground beef
- 8 oz (225 g) mushrooms, finely chopped
- 1/2 onion, finely chopped
- 2 cloves garlic, minced
- 1 tsp olive oil
- 1/2 tsp salt
- 1/4 tsp black pepper
- 1 tsp Italian seasoning
- 8 oz (240 ml) tomato sauce
- 4 oz (120 ml) low-sodium beef broth
- 8 oz (240 ml) cooked quinoa or brown rice
- 2 oz (60 g) shredded mozzarella cheese

Directions:

1. Preheat your oven to 375°F (190°C).
2. Cut the tops off the bell peppers and remove the seeds and membranes. Set aside.
3. In a large skillet, heat olive oil over medium heat. Add the onion and garlic, sauté until translucent.
4. Add the ground beef and cook until browned, breaking it into crumbles as it cooks. Drain any excess fat.

5. Stir in the chopped mushrooms, salt, black pepper, and Italian seasoning. Cook for another 5 minutes until the mushrooms release their moisture.
6. Add the cooked quinoa or brown rice to the meat and mushroom mixture, and stir until well combined.
7. Spoon the mixture into the hollowed-out bell peppers and place them in a baking dish.
8. Mix the tomato sauce and beef broth, then pour the mixture over the stuffed peppers.
9. Cover the baking dish with foil and bake for 30 minutes. Uncover and sprinkle the mozzarella cheese on top.
10. Bake for an additional 10 minutes, or until the cheese is melted and bubbly.
11. Serve the stuffed bell peppers with a side of salad or steamed vegetables.

**Nutritional Values:** Calories: 390 kcal | Fat: 12 g | Protein: 28 g | Carbs: 40 g | Net carbs: 30 g | Fiber: 10 g | Cholesterol: 70 mg | Sodium: 570 mg | Potassium: 980 mg

**Useful Tip:** You can customize this recipe by using different colored bell peppers for a vibrant presentation.

# Smoked Rabbit with Cranberry Chutney

Serving: 4 | Prep time: 15 minutes | Cook time: 90 minutes

## Ingredients:

- 24 oz (680 g) rabbit meat, cut into pieces
- 4 oz (115 g) hickory wood chips
- 2 tbsp olive oil
- 1 tsp smoked paprika
- 1/2 tsp salt
- 1/4 tsp black pepper
- 8 oz (240 g) cranberries
- 4 oz (120 ml) apple cider vinegar
- 4 oz (120 ml) water
- 2.25 oz (60 g) brown sugar
- 1/2 tsp ginger, minced

## Directions:

1. Soak the hickory wood chips in water for at least 30 minutes.
2. Preheat your smoker to 225°F (107°C) according to the manufacturer's instructions.
3. In a bowl, combine olive oil, smoked paprika, salt, and black pepper. Rub this mixture over the rabbit pieces.
4. Place the soaked wood chips in the smoker box and put the rabbit pieces on the grill grates. Smoke the rabbit for 60-90 minutes, or until it reaches an internal temperature of 165°F (74°C) and has a smoky flavor.
5. While the rabbit is smoking, prepare the cranberry chutney. In a saucepan, combine cranberries, apple cider vinegar, water, brown sugar, and minced ginger.
6. Cook over medium heat, stirring occasionally, until the cranberries burst and the chutney thickens, about 15-20 minutes.
7. Serve the smoked rabbit with a generous dollop of cranberry chutney.

**Nutritional Values:** Calories: 350 kcal | Fat: 10 g | Protein: 40 g | Carbs: 28 g | Net carbs: 24 g | Fiber: 4 g | Cholesterol: 130 mg | Sodium: 450 mg | Potassium: 760 mg

**Useful Tip:** For a milder smoke flavor, you can use fruitwood chips like apple or cherry instead of hickory.

# Quail and Broccoli Stir-Fry

Serving: 4 | Prep time: 15 minutes | Cook time: 20 minutes

Ingredients:

- 16 oz (450 g) quail, deboned and cut into bite-sized pieces
- 8 oz (225 g) broccoli florets
- 2 tbsp soy sauce
- 1 tbsp oyster sauce
- 1 tsp brown sugar
- 1/2 tsp ginger, minced
- 2 cloves garlic, minced
- 1/2 tsp cornstarch
- 2 tbsp vegetable oil
- 2 oz (60 ml) chicken broth
- 1/4 tsp red pepper flakes (adjust to taste)

Directions:

1. In a small bowl, whisk together soy sauce, oyster sauce, brown sugar, ginger, garlic, and cornstarch. Set aside.
2. Heat the vegetable oil in a wok or large skillet over high heat.
3. Add the quail pieces and stir-fry for about 3-4 minutes until they are no longer pink and have a light brown sear. Remove the quail from the pan and set aside.
4. In the same pan, add the broccoli florets and stir-fry for 2-3 minutes until they turn bright green and slightly tender.
5. Return the quail to the pan, pour the sauce mixture over the ingredients, and add the chicken broth. Stir-fry for an additional 2-3 minutes until everything is well-coated and heated through.
6. Sprinkle with red pepper flakes if you like a bit of heat.
7. Serve your quail and broccoli stir-fry over cooked brown rice or quinoa.

Nutritional Values: Calories: 280 kcal | Fat: 12 g | Protein: 30 g | Carbs: 12 g | Net carbs: 7 g | Fiber: 5 g | Cholesterol: 95 mg | Sodium: 660 mg | Potassium: 590 mg

Useful Tip: Don't overcook the quail as it can become tough; a quick sear is enough to keep it tender and flavorful.

# Mediterranean Lamb Kebabs

Serving: 4 | Prep time: 20 minutes | Cook time: 12 minutes

Ingredients:

- 16 oz (450 g) lean ground lamb
- 2 oz (60 ml) olive oil
- 2 cloves garlic, minced
- 1 tsp ground cumin
- 1 tsp ground coriander
- 1/2 tsp paprika
- 1/2 tsp salt
- 1/4 tsp black pepper
- Zest of 1 lemon
- Juice of 1 lemon
- 1 red onion, cut into chunks
- 1 red bell pepper, cut into chunks
- 1 yellow bell pepper, cut into chunks
- 8 wooden skewers, soaked in water for 30 minutes

Directions:

1. In a bowl, combine the ground lamb, half of the olive oil, minced garlic, ground cumin, ground coriander, paprika, salt, black pepper, lemon zest, and juice. Mix until well combined.
2. Divide the lamb mixture into 8 portions and shape each portion onto a wooden skewer to form kebabs.
3. Preheat your grill to medium-high heat (about 375°F or 190°C).
4. Thread the marinated lamb kebabs onto the soaked wooden skewers, alternating with chunks of red onion and bell pepper.
5. Brush the kebabs with the remaining olive oil to prevent sticking.
6. Grill the kebabs for about 4-6 minutes on each side, or until the lamb is cooked to your desired level of doneness and the vegetables are tender with a slight char.
7. Serve the Mediterranean Lamb Kebabs with your choice of Mediterranean side dishes, such as tzatziki and pita bread.

**Nutritional Values:** Calories: 320 kcal | Fat: 22 g | Protein: 25 g | Carbs: 8 g | Net carbs: 6 g | Fiber: 2 g | Cholesterol: 85 mg | Sodium: 460 mg | Potassium: 490 mg

**Useful Tip:** If you're using wooden skewers, soak them in water for at least 30 minutes to prevent them from burning on the grill.

# Lemon-Dijon Pork Chops

Serving: 4 | Prep time: 15 minutes | Cook time: 20 minutes

Ingredients:

- 4 boneless pork chops, 6 oz (170 g) each
- 2 tbsp olive oil
- 2 tbsp lemon juice
- 2 tbsp Dijon mustard
- 1 tsp honey
- 2 cloves garlic, minced
- 1 tsp dried thyme
- 1/2 tsp salt
- 1/4 tsp black pepper
- Zest of 1 lemon
- Fresh parsley for garnish (optional)

Directions:

1. In a bowl, whisk together the olive oil, lemon juice, Dijon mustard, honey, minced garlic, dried thyme, salt, black pepper, and lemon zest to make the marinade.
2. Place the pork chops in a resealable plastic bag or shallow dish and pour the marinade over them. Seal the bag or cover the dish and refrigerate for at least 30 minutes or marinate overnight for enhanced flavor.
3. Preheat your grill or skillet over medium-high heat.
4. Remove the pork chops from the marinade, allowing any excess to drip off.
5. Grill or pan-sear the pork chops for about 4-5 minutes per side, or until they reach an internal temperature of 145°F (63°C) and have a nice sear.
6. While grilling or searing, occasionally brush the pork chops with the remaining marinade.
7. Let the pork chops rest for a few minutes before serving. Garnish with fresh parsley if desired.

**Nutritional Values:** Calories: 290 kcal | Fat: 15 g | Protein: 30 g | Carbs: 4 g | Net carbs: 3 g | Fiber: 1 g | Cholesterol: 80 mg | Sodium: 420 mg | Potassium: 500 mg

# Chicken Piccata with Capers

Serving: 4 | Prep time: 15 minutes | Cook time: 20 minutes

## Ingredients:

- 4 boneless, skinless chicken breasts, 6 oz (170 g) each
- 4 oz (115 g) all-purpose flour
- 2 oz (60 ml) olive oil
- 2 oz (60 ml) chicken broth
- 2 oz (60 ml) lemon juice
- 2 oz (60 ml) brined capers, drained
- 2 cloves garlic, minced
- 2 tbsp unsalted butter
- 1/2 tsp salt
- 1/4 tsp black pepper
- Fresh parsley for garnish

## Directions:

1. Place the chicken breasts between two sheets of plastic wrap and gently pound them to an even thickness, about 1/2 inch (1.25 cm) thick.
2. In a shallow dish, mix the all-purpose flour with a pinch of salt and black pepper.
3. Dredge each chicken breast in the flour mixture, shaking off any excess.
4. In a large skillet, heat the olive oil over medium-high heat.
5. Add the chicken breasts and cook for about 3-4 minutes per side until they are golden brown and cooked through. Remove the chicken and set it aside.
6. In the same skillet, add the minced garlic and sauté for about 30 seconds until fragrant.
7. Pour in the chicken broth, and lemon juice. Bring to a simmer and cook for 3-4 minutes to reduce the sauce slightly.
8. Stir in the capers and unsalted butter, allowing the butter to melt into the sauce.
9. Return the cooked chicken to the skillet and simmer for an additional 2 minutes, allowing the chicken to heat through and absorb the flavors of the sauce.
10. Garnish with fresh parsley and serve your Chicken Piccata with capers over cooked pasta, rice, or steamed vegetables.

Nutritional Values: Calories: 320 kcal | Fat: 14 g | Protein: 28 g | Carbs: 15 g | Net carbs: 11 g | Fiber: 4 g | Cholesterol: 85 mg | Sodium: 640 mg | Potassium: 460 mg



# Thai Red Curry Turkey

Serving: 4 | Prep time: 15 minutes | Cook time: 20 minutes

## Ingredients:

- 16 oz (450 g) ground turkey
- 2 oz (60 g) red curry paste
- 14 oz (400 ml) coconut milk
- 2 oz (60 ml) chicken broth
- 1 red bell pepper, sliced
- 1 yellow bell pepper, sliced

- 6 oz (180 g) broccoli florets
- 2 tsp fish sauce
- 1 tsp brown sugar
- 1 tbsp vegetable oil
- 1/2 tsp salt
- 1/4 tsp black pepper
- Fresh cilantro for garnish
- Cooked rice or noodles for serving

Directions:

1. In a large skillet, heat the vegetable oil over medium-high heat.
2. Add the ground turkey and cook, breaking it into crumbles, until it's no longer pink and has a light brown sear.
3. Stir in the red curry paste and cook for 1-2 minutes to release its flavors.
4. Pour in the coconut milk and chicken broth, stirring to combine.
5. Add the red and yellow bell peppers, broccoli florets, fish sauce, and brown sugar. Stir well.
6. Cover and simmer for about 10-12 minutes, or until the vegetables are tender and the sauce thickens.
7. Season with salt and black pepper, adjusting to taste.
8. Serve your Thai Red Curry Turkey over cooked rice or noodles.
9. Garnish with fresh cilantro for a burst of color and flavor.

**Nutritional Values:** Calories: 350 kcal | Fat: 20 g | Protein: 24 g | Carbs: 20 g | Net carbs: 16 g | Fiber: 4 g | Cholesterol: 75 mg | Sodium: 730 mg | Potassium: 760 mg

**Useful Tip:** For extra heat, you can adjust the amount of red curry paste to suit your spice preference.

## Turkey and Spinach Stuffed Portobello Mushrooms

Serving: 4 | Prep time: 20 minutes | Cook time: 25 minutes

Ingredients:

- 4 large Portobello mushrooms
- 16 oz (450 g) ground turkey
- 8 oz (225 g) fresh spinach, chopped
- 4 oz (115 g) cream cheese
- 2 cloves garlic, minced
- 1/2 tsp dried oregano
- 1/2 tsp salt
- 1/4 tsp black pepper
- 2 oz (60 ml) chicken broth
- 2 oz (60 g) grated Parmesan cheese
- 2 oz (60 ml) olive oil
- Fresh basil leaves for garnish (optional)

Directions:

1. Preheat your oven to 375°F (190°C).
2. Clean the Portobello mushrooms and remove the stems. Place the mushrooms on a baking sheet, cap-side down.
3. In a skillet, heat 2 tablespoons of olive oil over medium heat. Add the chopped spinach and sauté until it wilts, about 3 minutes. Remove from the skillet and set aside.
4. In the same skillet, add the remaining olive oil and minced garlic. Sauté for about 30 seconds until fragrant.
5. Add the ground turkey, dried oregano, salt, and black pepper. Cook until the turkey is browned and cooked through.
6. Stir in the cream cheese until it melts and forms a creamy mixture.
7. Add the sautéed spinach and chicken broth to the turkey mixture. Cook for an additional 2-3 minutes until the mixture thickens slightly.
8. Fill each Portobello mushroom cap with the turkey and spinach mixture.

9. Sprinkle with grated Parmesan cheese and bake in the preheated oven for 20-25 minutes, or until the mushrooms are tender and the cheese is golden brown.
10. Garnish with fresh basil leaves if desired.

**Nutritional Values:** Calories: 350 kcal | Fat: 24 g | Protein: 28 g | Carbs: 10 g | Net carbs: 6 g | Fiber: 4 g | Cholesterol: 80 mg | Sodium: 610 mg | Potassium: 950 mg

**Useful Tip:** To make this recipe vegetarian, you can substitute the ground turkey with plant-based meat alternatives.

## Mediterranean-Style Veal Scaloppini

Serving: 4 | Prep time: 15 minutes | Cook time: 10 minutes

**Ingredients:**

- 16 oz (450 g) veal scaloppini
- 4 oz (115 g) all-purpose flour
- 2 oz (60 ml) olive oil
- 2 oz (60 ml) chicken broth
- 2 cloves garlic, minced
- 2 oz (60 ml) lemon juice
- 2 oz (60 g) cherry tomatoes, halved
- 2 oz (60 g) Kalamata olives, pitted and sliced
- 2 oz (60 g) artichoke hearts, quartered
- 1/2 tsp dried oregano
- 1/2 tsp salt
- 1/4 tsp black pepper
- Fresh basil leaves for garnish (optional)

**Directions:**

1. Lightly coat the veal scaloppini in all-purpose flour, shaking off any excess.
2. In a large skillet, heat the olive oil over medium-high heat.
3. Add the veal scaloppini and cook for about 2-3 minutes on each side until they are golden brown and cooked through. Remove the veal from the skillet and set it aside.
4. In the same skillet, add the minced garlic and sauté for about 30 seconds until fragrant.
5. Pour in the chicken broth and lemon juice. Bring to a simmer and cook for 2-3 minutes to reduce the sauce slightly.
6. Stir in the cherry tomatoes, Kalamata olives, artichoke hearts, dried oregano, salt, and black pepper. Cook for an additional 2-3 minutes until the tomatoes soften and the sauce thickens.
7. Return the cooked veal scaloppini to the skillet and simmer for an additional 2 minutes, allowing the veal to heat through and absorb the flavors of the sauce.
8. Garnish with fresh basil leaves if desired.

**Nutritional Values:** Calories: 350 kcal | Fat: 16 g | Protein: 28 g | Carbs: 12 g | Net carbs: 7 g | Fiber: 5 g | Cholesterol: 80 mg | Sodium: 720 mg | Potassium: 700 mg

**Useful Tip:** To keep the veal tender, be careful not to overcook it; it should be slightly pink in the center when done.

# Quail and Wild Mushroom Risotto

Serving: 4 | Prep time: 15 minutes | Cook time: 30 minutes

Ingredients:

- 4 semi-boneless quail (about 4 oz/115 g each)
- 8 oz (225 g) Arborio rice
- 6 oz (170 g) mixed wild mushrooms (such as shiitake, oyster, and porcini)
- 32 oz (960 ml) chicken broth
- 2 oz (60 g) shallots, finely chopped
- 2 cloves garlic, minced
- 2 oz (60 ml) olive oil
- 2 oz (60 g) Parmesan cheese, grated
- 1/2 tsp dried thyme
- 1/2 tsp salt
- 1/4 tsp black pepper
- Fresh parsley for garnish (optional)

Directions:

1. In a large skillet, heat the olive oil over medium heat.
2. Add the quail and cook for about 3-4 minutes on each side until they are golden brown and cooked through. Remove the quail from the skillet and set them aside.
3. In the same skillet, add the shallots and minced garlic. Sauté for about 2 minutes until they become translucent.
4. Stir in the Arborio rice and cook for another 2 minutes until the rice is well coated with the oil and slightly translucent.
5. Add the mixed wild mushrooms, dried thyme, salt, and black pepper. Stir well.
6. Begin adding the chicken broth one ladle at a time, stirring frequently and allowing the liquid to be absorbed before adding more.
7. Continue this process until the rice is creamy and tender but still slightly firm, about 18-20 minutes.
8. Stir in the grated Parmesan cheese and return the quail to the skillet, allowing them to heat through.
9. Garnish with fresh parsley if desired.

Nutritional Values: Calories: 400 kcal | Fat: 16 g | Protein: 32 g | Carbs: 30 g | Net carbs: 25 g | Fiber: 5 g | Cholesterol: 110 mg | Sodium: 820 mg | Potassium: 680 mg

Useful Tip: Keep the chicken broth warm in a separate pot to help maintain the temperature of the risotto.

# Grilled Quail with Rosemary and Garlic

Serving: 4 | Prep time: 10 minutes | Cook time: 20 minutes

Ingredients:

- 4 whole quails, about 4 oz (115 g) each
- 2 oz (60 ml) olive oil
- 4 cloves garlic, minced
- 1 oz (30 g) fresh rosemary, chopped
- 1 lemon, zested and juiced
- 1/2 tsp salt
- 1/4 tsp black pepper
- Lemon wedges for garnish
- Fresh rosemary sprigs for presentation

Directions:

1. In a bowl, combine the olive oil, minced garlic, chopped fresh rosemary, lemon zest, lemon juice, salt, and black pepper to create a marinade.
2. Place the quails in a large resealable bag or a shallow dish and pour the marinade over them. Ensure the quails are well-coated and refrigerate for at least 30 minutes, or ideally, overnight for better flavor absorption.
3. Preheat your grill to medium-high heat, about 375°F (190°C).
4. Remove the quails from the marinade and let any excess marinade drip off.
5. Place the quails on the grill, breast-side down, and grill for about 5-6 minutes on each side until they are cooked through and have a nice char.
6. Baste the quails with any remaining marinade while grilling.
7. Once done, remove the quails from the grill and let them rest for a few minutes before serving.
8. Garnish with lemon wedges and fresh rosemary sprigs for presentation.

**Nutritional Values:** Calories: 280 kcal | Fat: 18 g | Protein: 26 g | Carbs: 4 g | Net carbs: 2 g | Fiber: 2 g | Cholesterol: 95 mg | Sodium: 350 mg | Potassium: 460 mg

**Useful Tip:** To prevent the quails from drying out, be sure not to overcook them; quail should still have a slight pink hue in the center when done.

## Braised Veal Osso Buco

Serving: 4 | Prep time: 20 minutes | Cook time: 2 hours

Ingredients:

- 4 veal osso buco cuts, about 8 oz (225 g) each
- 2 oz (60 g) all-purpose flour
- 2 oz (60 ml) olive oil
- 4 oz (120 ml) beef broth
- 1 onion, finely chopped
- 2 carrots, finely chopped
- 2 celery stalks, finely chopped
- 4 cloves garlic, minced
- 1 can (14 oz/400 g) crushed tomatoes
- 2 oz (60 ml) tomato paste
- 1 oz (30 g) fresh parsley, chopped
- 1/2 tsp salt
- 1/4 tsp black pepper
- Zest of 1 lemon
- Grated Parmesan cheese for garnish (optional)
- Fresh parsley for garnish (optional)

Directions:

1. Dredge the veal osso buco in all-purpose flour, shaking off any excess.
2. In a large, oven-proof pot, heat the olive oil over medium-high heat.
3. Add the veal osso buco and sear for about 3-4 minutes on each side until they are golden brown. Remove the veal from the pot and set it aside.
4. In the same pot, add the chopped onion, carrots, and celery. Sauté for about 5 minutes until they soften.
5. Stir in the minced garlic and sauté for an additional 30 seconds until fragrant.
6. Add the crushed tomatoes, tomato paste, beef broth, fresh parsley, salt, black pepper, and lemon zest to the pot. Stir well.
7. Return the seared veal osso buco to the pot, nestling them into the sauce.

8. Cover the pot and place it in a preheated oven at 325°F (163°C). Braise for 1.5 to 2 hours until the veal is tender and easily pulls away from the bone.
9. Garnish with grated Parmesan cheese and fresh parsley if desired.

**Nutritional Values:** Calories: 450 kcal | Fat: 20 g | Protein: 30 g | Carbs: 30 g | Net carbs: 22 g | Fiber: 8 g | Cholesterol: 95 mg | Sodium: 780 mg | Potassium: 850 mg

**Useful Tip:** Serve the osso buco with gremolata, a mixture of lemon zest, garlic, and parsley, for an extra burst of flavor.

# VEGETARIAN RECIPES

## Butternut Squash and Sage Risotto

Serving: 4 | Prep time: 15 minutes | Cook time: 25 minutes

Ingredients:

- 8 oz (225 g) butternut squash, peeled, seeded, and diced
- 6 oz (170 g) Arborio rice
- 32 oz (960 ml) vegetable broth, warm
- 2 oz (60 g) shallots, finely chopped
- 2 cloves garlic, minced
- 2 oz (60 ml) olive oil
- 1 oz (30 g) vegan Parmesan cheese, grated
- 1 tbsp unsalted vegan butter
- 1 tsp fresh sage leaves, chopped
- Salt and black pepper to taste
- Fresh sage leaves for garnish

Directions:

1. In a large skillet, heat the olive oil over medium heat.
2. Add the chopped shallots and minced garlic. Sauté for about 2 minutes until they become translucent.
3. Stir in the Arborio rice and cook for another 2 minutes until the rice is well coated with the oil and slightly translucent.
4. Add the diced butternut squash and chopped sage leaves. Cook for 2-3 minutes, stirring occasionally.
5. Begin adding the warm vegetable broth one ladle at a time, stirring frequently and allowing the liquid to be absorbed before adding more.
6. Continue this process until the rice is creamy and tender but still slightly firm, about 18-20 minutes.
7. Stir in the grated Parmesan cheese and unsalted butter until well incorporated.
8. Season with salt and black pepper to taste.
9. Garnish with fresh sage leaves for presentation.

Nutritional Values: Calories: 350 kcal | Fat: 14 g | Protein: 6 g | Carbs: 50 g | Net carbs: 40 g | Fiber: 10 g | Cholesterol: 10 mg | Sodium: 780 mg | Potassium: 550 mg

Useful Tip: To save time, you can roast the diced butternut squash in the oven with a bit of olive oil, salt, and pepper while you prepare the rest of the risotto.

## Spicy Chickpea and Vegetable Curry

Serving: 4 | Prep time: 15 minutes | Cook time: 25 minutes

Ingredients:

- 14 oz (400 g) canned chickpeas, drained and rinsed
- 10 oz (280 g) cauliflower florets
- 7 oz (200 g) cherry tomatoes, halved
- 5 oz (140 g) baby spinach leaves
- 1 onion, finely chopped
- 2 cloves garlic, minced
- 1 oz (30 ml) olive oil
- 2 oz (60 ml) tomato paste
- 14 oz (400 ml) coconut milk

- 2 tsp curry powder
- 1/2 tsp turmeric powder
- 1/2 tsp cumin powder
- 1/2 tsp chili powder (adjust to taste)
- Salt and black pepper to taste
- Fresh cilantro leaves for garnish

## Directions:

1. In a large pan, heat the olive oil over medium heat.
2. Add the chopped onion and sauté until translucent, about 3 minutes.
3. Add the minced garlic, curry powder, turmeric powder, cumin powder, and chili powder. Sauté for 1-2 minutes until the spices are fragrant.
4. Stir in the tomato paste and cook for another 2 minutes.
5. Add the cauliflower florets and cherry tomatoes to the pan. Cook for 5 minutes, stirring occasionally.
6. Pour in the coconut milk and bring the mixture to a gentle simmer. Cook for 10-12 minutes until the cauliflower is tender.
7. Add the drained chickpeas and baby spinach leaves to the pan. Stir well and cook for an additional 3-4 minutes until the spinach wilts and the chickpeas are heated through.
8. Season with salt and black pepper to taste.
9. Garnish with fresh cilantro leaves before serving.

**Nutritional Values:** Calories: 350 kcal | Fat: 20 g | Protein: 10 g | Carbs: 35 g | Net carbs: 25 g | Fiber: 10 g | Cholesterol: 0 mg | Sodium: 600 mg | Potassium: 950 mg

**Useful Tip:** For a creamier curry, you can blend a portion of the cooked vegetables and coconut milk using an immersion blender before adding the chickpeas and spinach.

# Greek-Style Spanakopita Triangles

Serving: 4 | Prep time: 20 minutes | Cook time: 25 minutes

## Ingredients:

- 8 oz (225 g) fresh spinach, chopped
- 4 oz (115 g) vegan feta cheese, crumbled
- 2 oz (60 g) vegan ricotta cheese
- 1 oz (30 g) pine nuts, toasted
- 1/2 onion, finely chopped
- 2 cloves garlic, minced
- 2 tbsp olive oil
- 1/2 tsp dried oregano
- 1/2 tsp dried dill
- Salt and black pepper to taste
- 8 phyllo pastry sheets, thawed if frozen
- Olive oil spray

## Directions:

1. In a large skillet, heat 1 tablespoon of olive oil over medium heat. Add the chopped onion and minced garlic, and sauté until translucent, about 3 minutes.
2. Add the chopped spinach to the skillet and cook until wilted, about 2-3 minutes. Remove from heat and let it cool slightly.
3. In a mixing bowl, combine the wilted spinach, crumbled feta cheese, ricotta cheese, toasted pine nuts, dried oregano, dried dill, salt, and black pepper. Mix well.
4. Preheat the oven to 375°F (190°C).
5. Place one phyllo pastry sheet on a clean surface and brush it lightly with olive oil. Place another sheet on top and repeat the process until you have four layers.

6. Cut the layered phyllo into strips of equal width, about 3 inches wide.

7. Spoon a small amount of the spinach and cheese mixture onto the end of each strip.

8. Fold the phyllo over the filling to create a triangle shape. Continue folding in a triangle pattern until you reach the end of the strip.

9. Repeat the process with the remaining phyllo sheets and filling.

10. Place the triangles on a baking sheet lined with parchment paper. Lightly spray the tops with olive oil.

11. Bake in the preheated oven for 20-25 minutes or until golden brown and crispy.

12. Remove from the oven and let them cool slightly before serving.

**Nutritional Values:** Calories: 280 kcal | Fat: 18 g | Protein: 9 g | Carbs: 23 g | Net carbs: 20 g | Fiber: 3 g | Cholesterol: 25 mg | Sodium: 400 mg | Potassium: 350 mg

**Useful Tip:** If you have any leftover phyllo sheets, keep them covered with a damp cloth to prevent drying out while working with the individual sheets.

## Eggplant Parmesan with Marinara Sauce

Serving: 4 | Prep time: 20 minutes | Cook time: 40 minutes

### Ingredients:

- 2 medium-sized eggplants (about 24 oz or 680 g), sliced into 1/2-inch rounds
- 14 oz (400 g) marinara sauce
- 8 oz (225 g) vegan mozzarella cheese, shredded
- 2 oz (60 g) grated vegan Parmesan cheese
- 4 oz (120 ml) olive oil

- 2 large eggs
- 4 oz (115 g) breadcrumbs
- 2 oz (60 g) all-purpose flour
- 2 tsp dried oregano
- 1 tsp garlic powder
- Salt and black pepper to taste
- Fresh basil leaves for garnish

### Directions:

1. Preheat your oven to 375°F (190°C).

2. In a shallow dish, mix the breadcrumbs, dried oregano, garlic powder, salt, and black pepper.

3. In another dish, place the all-purpose flour.

4. In a third dish, beat the eggs.

5. Dredge each eggplant slice in the flour, dip in the beaten eggs, and coat with the breadcrumb mixture, ensuring an even coating.

6. In a large skillet, heat the olive oil over medium-high heat. Fry the breaded eggplant slices until they turn golden brown, about 2-3 minutes per side. Place them on paper towels to remove excess oil.

7. In a baking dish, spread a thin layer of marinara sauce.

8. Place a layer of fried eggplant slices on top of the sauce.

9. Sprinkle some mozzarella and Parmesan cheese over the eggplant.

10. Repeat the layers until all the eggplant is used, finishing with a layer of sauce and cheese on top.

11. Bake in the preheated oven for 20-25 minutes until the cheese is bubbly and golden.

12. Garnish with fresh basil leaves before serving.

**Nutritional Values:** Calories: 450 kcal | Fat: 28 g | Protein: 20 g | Carbs: 30 g | Net carbs: 20 g | Fiber: 10 g | Cholesterol: 90 mg | Sodium: 900 mg | Potassium: 900 mg

Useful Tip: For a lighter version, you can also bake the eggplant slices instead of frying them for a healthier dish.

## Sweet Potato and Black Bean Enchiladas

Serving: 4 | Prep time: 20 minutes | Cook time: 35 minutes

Ingredients:

- 2 medium sweet potatoes (about 16 oz or 450 g), peeled and diced
- 15 oz (425 g) canned black beans, drained and rinsed
- 4 oz (115 g) shredded vegan cheddar cheese
- 8 small corn tortillas
- 4 oz (120 ml) enchilada sauce
- 4 oz (120 ml) plain Greek yogurt
- 1 tsp chili powder
- 1/2 tsp cumin
- 1/2 tsp paprika
- Salt and black pepper to taste
- Chopped fresh cilantro for garnish

Directions:

1. Preheat your oven to 375°F (190°C).
2. Place the diced sweet potatoes in a microwave-safe bowl, cover with a damp paper towel, and microwave for 5-7 minutes, or until tender.
3. In a large mixing bowl, combine the cooked sweet potatoes, black beans, chili powder, cumin, paprika, salt, and black pepper. Mash and mix until well combined.
4. Warm the corn tortillas in the microwave for about 30 seconds to make them pliable.
5. Lay out each tortilla and divide the sweet potato and black bean mixture equally among them. Roll them up tightly and place them seam side down in a baking dish.
6. Pour the enchilada sauce over the top of the rolled tortillas.
7. Sprinkle the shredded cheddar cheese on top.
8. Bake in the preheated oven for 20-25 minutes or until the cheese is melted and bubbly.
9. Serve with a dollop of Greek yogurt and garnish with chopped cilantro.

Nutritional Values: Calories: 380 kcal | Fat: 12 g | Protein: 17 g | Carbs: 55 g | Net carbs: 43 g | Fiber: 12 g | Cholesterol: 30 mg | Sodium: 560 mg | Potassium: 700 mg

Useful Tip: You can customize these enchiladas by adding diced avocado, sliced jalapeños, or a squeeze of lime for extra flavor. You can replace Greek yogurt with: almond milk yogurt, cashew yogurt, and coconut yogurt.

## Quinoa-Stuffed Acorn Squash

Serving: 4 | Prep time: 15 minutes | Cook time: 45 minutes

Ingredients:

- 2 acorn squash, halved and seeds removed
- 6 oz (170 g) quinoa
- 16 oz (480 ml) vegetable broth
- 4 oz (115 g) chopped kale
- 2 oz (55 g) dried cranberries
- 2 oz (55 g) chopped pecans
- 2 tbsp olive oil
- 1 tsp ground cinnamon
- 1/2 tsp ground nutmeg
- Salt and black pepper to taste
- Fresh parsley for garnish

**Directions:**

1. Preheat your oven to 375°F (190°C).
2. Brush the inside of the acorn squash halves with olive oil and season with a pinch of salt and black pepper.
3. Place the squash halves, cut side down, on a baking sheet and roast in the preheated oven for 25-30 minutes, or until they're tender and easily pierced with a fork.
4. While the squash is roasting, rinse the quinoa under cold water and drain.
5. In a medium saucepan, combine the rinsed quinoa and vegetable broth. Bring to a boil, then reduce the heat, cover, and simmer for 15 minutes or until the quinoa is cooked and the liquid is absorbed.
6. In a large bowl, combine the cooked quinoa, chopped kale, dried cranberries, chopped pecans, ground cinnamon, ground nutmeg, and a pinch of salt and black pepper.
7. When the squash is ready, remove it from the oven and carefully turn the halves over.
8. Fill each squash half with the quinoa mixture.
9. Return the filled squash to the oven and bake for an additional 15 minutes.
10. Garnish with fresh parsley before serving.

**Nutritional Values:** Calories: 420 kcal | Fat: 16 g | Protein: 10 g | Carbs: 65 g | Net carbs: 55 g | Fiber: 10 g | Cholesterol: 0 mg | Sodium: 320 mg | Potassium: 1130 mg

**Useful Tip:** Drizzle with honey or maple syrup for a touch of sweetness if desired.

# Mediterranean Ratatouille

Serving: 4 | Prep time: 15 minutes | Cook time: 30 minutes

**Ingredients:**

- 1 large eggplant (12 oz / 340 g), diced
- 2 zucchinis (12 oz / 340 g), diced
- 2 bell peppers (8 oz / 225 g), diced
- 1 onion (4 oz / 115 g), diced
- 3 cloves garlic, minced
- 1 can (14 oz / 400 g) diced tomatoes
- 2 tbsp olive oil
- 1 tsp dried basil
- 1 tsp dried oregano
- Salt and black pepper to taste
- Fresh basil leaves for garnish

**Directions:**

1. Heat the olive oil in a large skillet over medium heat.
2. Add the diced onion and sauté for 2-3 minutes until it becomes translucent.
3. Stir in the minced garlic and sauté for another 30 seconds until fragrant.
4. Add the diced eggplant, zucchini, and bell peppers to the skillet and cook for 10 minutes, stirring occasionally, until they start to soften.
5. Pour in the canned diced tomatoes and add the dried basil, dried oregano, salt, and black pepper. Stir to combine.
6. Reduce the heat to low, cover the skillet, and let the ratatouille simmer for an additional 15 minutes, or until all the vegetables are tender and the flavors have melded together.
7. Taste and adjust the seasoning if needed.
8. Garnish with fresh basil leaves before serving.

Nutritional Values: Calories: 150 kcal | Fat: 7 g | Protein: 3 g | Carbs: 22 g | Net carbs: 15 g | Fiber: 7 g | Cholesterol: 0 mg | Sodium: 400 mg | Potassium: 820 mg

Useful Tip: This dish can be served hot as a side dish or cold as a refreshing salad.

## Caprese Zucchini Noodles with Pesto

Serving: 4 | Prep time: 20 minutes | Cook time: 5 minutes

Ingredients:

- 4 medium zucchinis (24 oz / 680 g), spiralized into noodles
- 8 oz (225 g) cherry tomatoes, halved
- 4 oz (115 g) fresh vegan mozzarella balls, small
- 4 oz (120 ml) pesto sauce
- 2 tbsp extra-virgin olive oil
- 2 tbsp balsamic vinegar
- Fresh basil leaves for garnish
- Salt and black pepper to taste

Directions:

1. In a large mixing bowl, combine the zucchini noodles, halved cherry tomatoes, and fresh mozzarella balls.
2. In a small bowl, whisk together the pesto sauce, extra-virgin olive oil, and balsamic vinegar.
3. Drizzle the pesto mixture over the zucchini noodles and toss gently to coat all ingredients.
4. Season with salt and black pepper to taste.
5. Garnish with fresh basil leaves for an extra burst of flavor.

Nutritional Values: Calories: 280 kcal | Fat: 22 g | Protein: 10 g | Carbs: 12 g | Net carbs: 6 g | Fiber: 6 g | Cholesterol: 20 mg | Sodium: 390 mg | Potassium: 460 mg

Useful Tip: If you don't have a spiralizer, you can use a vegetable peeler to create zucchini ribbons instead.

## Mushroom and Spinach Stuffed Portobello Mushrooms

Serving: 4 | Prep time: 15 minutes | Cook time: 25 minutes

Ingredients:

- 4 large Portobello mushrooms (20 oz / 570 g)
- 10 oz (280 g) cremini mushrooms, finely chopped
- 2 oz (60 g) fresh spinach, chopped
- 2 oz (55 g) grated vegan Parmesan cheese
- 4 oz (115 g) vegan cream cheese
- 2 cloves garlic, minced
- 2 tbsp olive oil
- 1 tsp balsamic vinegar
- 1/2 tsp dried thyme
- Salt and black pepper to taste

Directions:

1. Preheat your oven to 375°F (190°C).
2. Remove the stems from the Portobello mushrooms and scrape out the gills to create a cavity. Brush the mushroom caps with olive oil and place them on a baking sheet.
3. In a skillet, heat 2 tablespoons of olive oil over medium heat. Add the chopped cremini mushrooms, garlic, and dried thyme. Sauté for about 5 minutes until the mushrooms are tender.
4. Stir in the chopped spinach and cook for an additional 2 minutes until wilted.

5. Remove the skillet from heat and let it cool slightly. Then, stir in the grated Parmesan cheese and cream cheese until well combined.
6. Season the mushroom and spinach mixture with salt and black pepper.
7. Carefully fill the Portobello mushroom caps with the stuffing mixture.
8. Drizzle a bit of balsamic vinegar over each stuffed mushroom.
9. Bake in the preheated oven for 20-25 minutes or until the mushrooms are tender and the stuffing is golden brown.
10. Serve hot and enjoy!

**Nutritional Values:** Calories: 240 kcal | Fat: 18 g | Protein: 11 g | Carbs: 11 g | Net carbs: 6 g | Fiber: 5 g | Cholesterol: 40 mg | Sodium: 340 mg | Potassium: 820 mg

**Useful Tip:** You can add a sprinkle of fresh parsley or extra Parmesan cheese for extra flavor and presentation.

# Spinach and Feta Stuffed Bell Peppers

Serving: 4 | Prep time: 20 minutes | Cook time: 30 minutes

## Ingredients:

- 4 large bell peppers (20 oz / 570 g)
- 8 oz (225 g) fresh spinach, chopped
- 4 oz (115 g) crumbled vegan feta cheese
- 4 oz (115 g) cooked quinoa
- 4 oz (115 g) diced tomatoes
- 2 cloves garlic, minced
- 1/2 tsp dried oregano
- Salt and black pepper to taste
- 2 tbsp olive oil
- Fresh basil leaves for garnish

## Directions:

1. Preheat your oven to 375°F (190°C).
2. Cut the tops off the bell peppers, remove the seeds and membranes, and set them aside.
3. In a large skillet, heat 2 tablespoons of olive oil over medium heat. Add minced garlic and sauté for about 1 minute until fragrant.
4. Add the chopped spinach to the skillet and cook for 3-4 minutes until wilted.
5. In a mixing bowl, combine the cooked quinoa, diced tomatoes, crumbled feta cheese, dried oregano, and the sautéed spinach. Mix everything together and season with salt and black pepper to taste.
6. Stuff each bell pepper with the spinach, quinoa, and feta mixture, pressing it down gently as you go.
7. Place the stuffed bell peppers in a baking dish, and cover the dish with foil.
8. Bake in the preheated oven for 20-25 minutes, removing the foil for the last 10 minutes to allow the tops to brown.
9. Garnish with fresh basil leaves.
10. Serve hot and enjoy!

**Nutritional Values:** Calories: 260 kcal | Fat: 14 g | Protein: 11 g | Carbs: 24 g | Net carbs: 17 g | Fiber: 7 g | Cholesterol: 30 mg | Sodium: 510 mg | Potassium: 890 mg

**Useful Tip:** You can customize this recipe by adding your favorite vegetables or spices to the stuffing mixture for extra flavor.

# Grilled Vegetable Tacos with Avocado Cream

Serving: 4 | Prep time: 15 minutes | Cook time: 15 minutes

Ingredients:

- 8 small corn tortillas
- 1 zucchini (8 oz / 225 g), sliced
- 1 yellow bell pepper (8 oz / 225 g), sliced
- 1 red onion (4 oz / 115 g), sliced into rings
- 4 oz (115 g) cherry tomatoes
- 1 ear of corn, husked
- 1 tbsp olive oil
- Salt and black pepper to taste

For the Avocado Cream:

- 1 ripe avocado (8 oz / 225 g)
- 4 oz (115 g) Greek yogurt
- Juice of 1 lime
- 1 clove garlic, minced
- Salt and black pepper to taste

Directions:

1. Preheat your grill to medium-high heat (around 400°F/200°C).
2. Brush the sliced zucchini, yellow bell pepper, red onion rings, cherry tomatoes, and ear of corn with olive oil. Season with salt and black pepper.
3. Place the vegetables on the grill. Grill the zucchini, bell pepper, and onion for about 5-7 minutes per side until charred and tender. Grill the corn for about 10 minutes, turning occasionally, until it's lightly charred. Remove the vegetables from the grill when done.
4. While the corn is still warm, carefully cut the kernels from the cob.
5. In a bowl, combine the avocado, Greek yogurt, lime juice, minced garlic, salt, and black pepper. Mash and mix until smooth to create the avocado cream.
6. Warm the corn tortillas on the grill for about 30 seconds per side.
7. To assemble the tacos, spread a spoonful of avocado cream on each tortilla. Add grilled zucchini, bell pepper, onion, cherry tomatoes, and corn kernels.
8. Serve the tacos hot and enjoy!

Nutritional Values: Calories: 275 kcal | Fat: 9 g | Protein: 7 g | Carbs: 46 g | Net carbs: 30 g | Fiber: 16 g | Cholesterol: 3 mg | Sodium: 190 mg | Potassium: 830 mg

Useful Tip: You can customize your grilled vegetable tacos with your favorite toppings like shredded cheese, fresh cilantro, or a drizzle of hot sauce. You can replace Greek yogurt with: almond milk yogurt, cashew yogurt, and coconut yogurt.

# Spaghetti Aglio e Olio with Roasted Tomatoes

Serving: 4 | Prep time: 10 minutes | Cook time: 20 minutes

Ingredients:

- 12 oz (340 g) whole wheat spaghetti
- 1 pint (16 oz / 450 g) cherry tomatoes
- 4 cloves garlic, thinly sliced
- 4 oz (115 g) extra virgin olive oil
- 1 tsp red pepper flakes (adjust to your spice preference)
- Salt and black pepper to taste
- 1 oz (28 g) fresh parsley, chopped

- Zest of 1 lemon
- Grated Parmesan cheese for serving (optional)

## Directions:

1. Preheat your oven to 425°F (220°C).
2. Place the cherry tomatoes on a baking sheet, drizzle with a bit of olive oil, and season with salt and black pepper. Roast them in the preheated oven for 15-20 minutes until they start to blister and burst.
3. While the tomatoes are roasting, cook the whole wheat spaghetti according to the package instructions until al dente. Drain and set aside.
4. In a large skillet, heat the remaining olive oil over medium-low heat. Add the sliced garlic and red pepper flakes. Sauté for about 2-3 minutes, or until the garlic is fragrant but not browned.
5. Add the cooked spaghetti to the skillet, tossing it in the garlic-infused oil.
6. Once the roasted tomatoes are done, add them to the skillet and gently mix them in with the pasta.
7. Remove from heat, then stir in the chopped fresh parsley and lemon zest.
8. Season with additional salt, black pepper, and red pepper flakes as desired.
9. Serve hot, with a sprinkle of grated Parmesan cheese if you like.

**Nutritional Values:** Calories: 450 kcal | Fat: 24 g | Protein: 9 g | Carbs: 50 g | Net carbs: 44 g | Fiber: 6 g | Cholesterol: 0 mg | Sodium: 100 mg | Potassium: 350 mg

**Useful Tip:** You can adjust the level of spice in your dish by increasing or decreasing the amount of red pepper flakes.

## Lentil and Vegetable Stir-Fry

Serving: 4 | Prep time: 15 minutes | Cook time: 20 minutes

## Ingredients:

- 8 oz (225 g) green or brown lentils
- 1.5 lbs (680 g) mixed vegetables (bell peppers, broccoli, carrots, snow peas, etc.), sliced
- 2 tbsp olive oil
- 3 cloves garlic, minced
- 1-inch piece (2.5 cm) fresh ginger, minced
- 2 oz (60 ml) low-sodium soy sauce
- 2 tbsp rice vinegar
- 1 tbsp honey or maple syrup
- 1 tsp red pepper flakes (adjust to your spice preference)
- Salt and black pepper to taste
- Chopped green onions and sesame seeds for garnish
- Cooked brown rice or quinoa for serving (optional)

## Directions:

1. Cook the lentils according to the package instructions. Drain and set aside.
2. In a large wok or skillet, heat the olive oil over medium-high heat.
3. Add the minced garlic and ginger, and stir-fry for about 1 minute until fragrant.
4. Add the sliced mixed vegetables to the wok and stir-fry for 5-7 minutes until they are crisp-tender and slightly caramelized.
5. In a small bowl, whisk together the soy sauce, rice vinegar, honey or maple syrup, and red pepper flakes.

6. Pour the sauce over the stir-fried vegetables and add the cooked lentils. Toss to combine and coat everything with the sauce.
7. Season with salt and black pepper to taste.
8. Cook for an additional 2-3 minutes to heat everything through.
9. Serve hot, garnished with chopped green onions and sesame seeds. You can also serve it over cooked brown rice or quinoa if you prefer.

**Nutritional Values:** Calories: 320 kcal | Fat: 7 g | Protein: 15 g | Carbs: 50 g | Net carbs: 35 g | Fiber: 15 g | Cholesterol: 0 mg | Sodium: 800 mg | Potassium: 760 mg

**Useful Tip:** Adjust the spice level by increasing or decreasing the amount of red pepper flakes in the sauce.

# Ratatouille Stuffed Tomatoes

Serving: 4 | Prep time: 15 minutes | Cook time: 35 minutes

**Ingredients:**

- 4 large tomatoes
- 4 oz (115 g) zucchini, diced
- 4 oz (115 g) eggplant, diced
- 4 oz (115 g) red bell pepper, diced
- 2 oz (60 g) onion, diced
- 2 cloves garlic, minced
- 2 tbsp olive oil
- 1 tsp dried thyme
- 1 tsp dried basil
- Salt and black pepper to taste
- 2 oz (60 ml) tomato sauce
- 2 tbsp balsamic vinegar
- Fresh basil leaves for garnish

**Directions:**

1. Preheat the oven to 375°F (190°C).
2. Slice off the top of each tomato and carefully scoop out the pulp and seeds, leaving a tomato shell. Season the insides of the tomatoes with a pinch of salt.
3. In a large skillet, heat the olive oil over medium heat.
4. Add the diced onion, garlic, and a pinch of salt. Sauté for 2-3 minutes until the onion becomes translucent.
5. Add the diced zucchini, eggplant, and red bell pepper to the skillet. Sauté for 5-7 minutes until the vegetables are tender.
6. Stir in the dried thyme and basil, then season with salt and black pepper to taste.
7. Add the tomato sauce and balsamic vinegar to the skillet. Cook for an additional 2-3 minutes until the mixture thickens slightly.
8. Fill each hollowed tomato with the ratatouille mixture, packing it gently.
9. Place the stuffed tomatoes in a baking dish, cover with aluminum foil, and bake in the preheated oven for 20 minutes.
10. Remove the foil and bake for an additional 10 minutes or until the tomato shells are tender and slightly roasted.
11. Garnish with fresh basil leaves before serving.

**Nutritional Values:** Calories: 123 kcal | Fat: 6 g | Protein: 2 g | Carbs: 16 g | Net carbs: 10 g | Fiber: 6 g | Cholesterol: 0 mg | Sodium: 150 mg | Potassium: 647 mg

**Useful Tip:** If you have any leftover ratatouille mixture, it makes a great side dish or can be served over pasta.

# SOUPS

## Minestrone Soup with Mixed Vegetables and Cannellini Beans

Serving: 4 | Prep time: 15 minutes | Cook time: 30 minutes

Ingredients:

- 1 oz (28 g) olive oil
- 2 oz (60 g) onion, chopped
- 2 cloves garlic, minced
- 2 oz (60 g) carrots, diced
- 2 oz (60 g) celery, diced
- 2 oz (60 g) zucchini, diced
- 2 oz (60 g) green beans, cut into bite-sized pieces
- 1 oz (28 g) tomato paste
- 1 tsp dried basil
- 1 tsp dried oregano
- 1/2 tsp salt
- 1/4 tsp black pepper
- 1 can (14 oz / 400 g) diced tomatoes
- 32 oz (960 ml) vegetable broth
- 1 can (14 oz / 400 g) cannellini beans, drained and rinsed
- 2 oz (60 g) small pasta (e.g., ditalini or macaroni)
- 2 oz (60 g) green peas (fresh or frozen)
- 2 oz (60 g) fresh spinach leaves
- Grated Parmesan cheese for garnish

Directions:

1. In a large pot, heat the olive oil over medium heat.
2. Add the chopped onion and minced garlic. Sauté for 2-3 minutes until fragrant and the onion turns translucent.
3. Stir in the diced carrots, celery, zucchini, and green beans. Sauté for an additional 5 minutes.
4. Add the tomato paste, dried basil, dried oregano, salt, and black pepper. Cook for 2 minutes while stirring.
5. Pour in the diced tomatoes and vegetable broth. Bring the mixture to a boil.
6. Reduce the heat and let the soup simmer for 10 minutes.
7. Stir in the cannellini beans, small pasta, and green peas. Continue to simmer for 10-12 minutes until the pasta is tender.
8. Just before serving, add the fresh spinach leaves and cook until they wilt, about 2 minutes.
9. Taste and adjust the seasoning if needed.
10. Serve hot, garnished with grated Parmesan cheese.

**Nutritional Values:** Calories: 215 kcal | Fat: 6 g | Protein: 8 g | Carbs: 34 g | Net carbs: 16 g | Fiber: 18 g | Cholesterol: 0 mg | Sodium: 1078 mg | Potassium: 732 mg

**Useful Tip:** You can customize this minestrone soup by adding other vegetables like bell peppers, corn, or potatoes.

# Moroccan Lentil Soup with Spiced Tomato Broth

Serving: 4 | Prep time: 10 minutes | Cook time: 25 minutes

Ingredients:

- 1 oz (28 g) olive oil
- 2 oz (60 g) onion, chopped
- 2 cloves garlic, minced
- 1 oz (28 g) carrots, diced
- 1 oz (28 g) celery, diced
- 1 oz (28 g) red bell pepper, diced
- 1 tsp ground cumin
- 1/2 tsp ground coriander
- 1/2 tsp ground paprika
- 1/2 tsp ground cinnamon
- 1/2 tsp ground turmeric
- 1/4 tsp cayenne pepper (adjust to taste)
- 7 oz (200 g) dried red lentils, rinsed and drained
- 1 can (14 oz / 400 g) diced tomatoes
- 32 oz (960 ml) vegetable broth
- 2 oz (60 g) kale, chopped
- Juice of 1 lemon
- Salt and pepper to taste
- Fresh cilantro leaves for garnish
- Plain yogurt (optional, for garnish)

Directions:

1. In a large pot, heat the olive oil over medium heat.
2. Add the chopped onion and minced garlic. Sauté for 2-3 minutes until fragrant and the onion turns translucent.
3. Stir in the diced carrots, celery, and red bell pepper. Sauté for an additional 5 minutes.
4. Add the ground cumin, ground coriander, ground paprika, ground cinnamon, ground turmeric, and cayenne pepper. Cook for 2 minutes while stirring.
5. Pour in the rinsed red lentils, diced tomatoes, and vegetable broth. Bring the mixture to a boil.
6. Reduce the heat and let the soup simmer for 15-20 minutes, or until the lentils are tender.
7. Stir in the chopped kale and cook until wilted, about 2 minutes.
8. Add lemon juice and season with salt and pepper to taste.
9. Serve hot, garnished with fresh cilantro leaves and a dollop of plain yogurt if desired.

**Nutritional Values:** Calories: 218 kcal | Fat: 6 g | Protein: 10 g | Carbs: 34 g | Net carbs: 14 g | Fiber: 20 g | Cholesterol: 0 mg | Sodium: 980 mg | Potassium: 646 mg

**Useful Tip:** Adjust the level of spiciness by varying the amount of cayenne pepper, or omit it for a milder flavor.

# Creamy Broccoli and Cheddar Soup

Serving: 4 | Prep time: 15 minutes | Cook time: 30 minutes

Ingredients:

- 1 oz (28 g) butter
- 1 oz (28 g) onion, chopped
- 1 oz (28 g) carrots, diced
- 1 oz (28 g) celery, diced
- 2 cloves garlic, minced
- 1 lb (450 g) fresh broccoli, stems and florets, chopped
- 32 oz (960 ml) vegetable broth
- 4 oz (115 g) sharp cheddar cheese, grated
- 8 oz (240 ml) whole milk

- 2 oz (60 g) all-purpose flour
- 2 oz (60 ml) heavy cream
- Salt and pepper to taste
- Pinch of nutmeg (optional)
- Fresh chives for garnish (optional)

## Directions:

1. In a large pot, melt the butter over medium heat.
2. Add chopped onions, diced carrots, and celery. Sauté for 5 minutes until softened.
3. Stir in minced garlic and sauté for another minute.
4. Add the chopped broccoli, vegetable broth, salt, and pepper. Bring to a boil, then reduce the heat and simmer for 15-20 minutes, or until the broccoli is tender.
5. Using an immersion blender, puree the soup until smooth. Alternatively, transfer it in batches to a blender.
6. In a separate saucepan, prepare a roux by melting 1 oz of butter over medium heat. Stir in the flour and cook for 2-3 minutes while whisking continuously.
7. Slowly whisk in the milk, then add the roux mixture to the soup. Stir well.
8. Gradually add the grated cheddar cheese and heavy cream, continuously stirring until the cheese is fully melted and the soup is creamy.
9. Season with a pinch of nutmeg (if desired) and adjust the salt and pepper to taste.
10. Serve hot, garnished with fresh chives.

**Nutritional Values:** Calories: 382 kcal | Fat: 25 g | Protein: 12 g | Carbs: 30 g | Net carbs: 22 g | Fiber: 8 g | Cholesterol: 75 mg | Sodium: 820 mg | Potassium: 635 mg

**Useful Tip:** Be cautious not to boil the soup after adding the cheese to prevent it from becoming grainy.

# Thai-Inspired Coconut Curry Soup with Tofu

Serving: 4 | Prep time: 15 minutes | Cook time: 30 minutes

## Ingredients:

- 8 oz (225 g) extra-firm tofu, cubed
- 2 oz (60 g) rice noodles
- 1 oz (30 g) red bell pepper, thinly sliced
- 1 oz (30 g) yellow bell pepper, thinly sliced
- 1 oz (30 g) snow peas, trimmed
- 1 oz (30 g) shiitake mushrooms, sliced
- 1 can (13.5 oz / 400 ml) coconut milk
- 32 oz (960 ml) vegetable broth
- 2 tbsp Thai red curry paste
- 1 oz (30 g) fresh cilantro, chopped
- 2 tbsp soy sauce
- 1 tbsp lime juice
- 1 tsp sesame oil
- 1 tsp vegetable oil
- Salt to taste
- Lime wedges and additional cilantro for garnish (optional)

## Directions:

1. In a large pot, heat the vegetable oil over medium-high heat.
2. Add the tofu cubes and cook until they are golden and crispy on all sides. Remove from the pot and set aside.
3. In the same pot, add the red curry paste and cook for a minute.
4. Pour in the coconut milk and vegetable broth, stirring until well combined.
5. Bring the mixture to a gentle boil, then reduce the heat and let it simmer for 10 minutes.

6.  Add the rice noodles, red bell pepper, yellow bell pepper, snow peas, and shiitake mushrooms to the pot. Simmer until the noodles are tender (usually about 5 minutes).
7.  Stir in the soy sauce, lime juice, and sesame oil.
8.  Season with salt to taste.
9.  Add the crispy tofu back to the pot.
10. Serve hot, garnished with fresh cilantro and lime wedges, if desired.

**Nutritional Values:** Calories: 332 kcal | Fat: 21 g | Protein: 9 g | Carbs: 29 g | Net carbs: 15 g | Fiber: 14 g | Cholesterol: 0 mg | Sodium: 1401 mg | Potassium: 480 mg

**Useful Tip:** Adjust the amount of Thai red curry paste based on your preferred level of spiciness.

## Butternut Squash and Apple Soup with Cinnamon

Serving: 4 | Prep time: 15 minutes | Cook time: 40 minutes

**Ingredients:**

- 12 oz (340 g) butternut squash, peeled, seeded, and diced
- 2 medium apples (such as Granny Smith or Honeycrisp), peeled, cored, and diced
- 1 small onion, chopped
- 32 oz (960 ml) vegetable broth
- 8 oz (240 ml) unsweetened almond milk
- 2 tsp olive oil
- 1 tsp ground cinnamon
- 1/2 tsp ground nutmeg
- Salt and pepper to taste
- Fresh chives for garnish (optional)

**Directions:**

1.  In a large pot, heat the olive oil over medium heat. Add the chopped onion and sauté until translucent.
2.  Add the diced butternut squash, apples, ground cinnamon, and ground nutmeg. Cook for 5 minutes, stirring occasionally.
3.  Pour in the vegetable broth and bring the mixture to a boil. Reduce heat and let it simmer for about 25-30 minutes, or until the butternut squash is tender.
4.  Using an immersion blender or countertop blender, purée the soup until smooth.
5.  Return the soup to the pot and stir in the almond milk. Heat the soup over low heat until it's warm.
6.  Season the soup with salt and pepper to taste.
7.  Serve the soup hot, garnished with fresh chives if desired.

**Nutritional Values:** Calories: 250 kcal | Fat: 10 g | Protein: 11 g | Carbs: 30 g | Net carbs: 18 g | Fiber: 12 g | Cholesterol: 0 mg | Sodium: 850 mg | Potassium: 440 mg

**Useful Tip:** Adjust the level of cinnamon and nutmeg to your taste preference; you can also add a touch of honey for sweetness if desired.

# Creamy Tomato Basil Soup with Garlic Croutons

Serving: 4 | Prep time: 15 minutes | Cook time: 30 minutes

Ingredients:

- 28 oz (800 g) canned crushed tomatoes
- 1 onion, chopped
- 2 cloves garlic, minced
- 2 oz (60 ml) heavy cream
- 32 oz (960 ml) vegetable broth
- 2 oz (60 ml) fresh basil leaves, chopped
- 2 tbsp olive oil
- 2 oz (50 g) stale bread, cut into cubes
- 1/2 tsp dried oregano
- Salt and pepper to taste

Directions:

1. In a large pot, heat the olive oil over medium heat. Add the chopped onion and cook until translucent.
2. Stir in the minced garlic and cook for another minute until fragrant.
3. Add the canned crushed tomatoes, vegetable broth, and dried oregano. Season with salt and pepper. Bring to a boil, then reduce the heat and simmer for 15-20 minutes.
4. Use an immersion blender or countertop blender to purée the soup until smooth. Return it to the pot.
5. Stir in the heavy cream and chopped fresh basil. Simmer for an additional 5 minutes.
6. While the soup is simmering, prepare the garlic croutons. In a separate pan, heat a little olive oil over medium heat. Add the bread cubes and toast until they are golden and crispy, then remove from heat.
7. Serve the creamy tomato basil soup hot, garnished with garlic croutons.

**Nutritional Values:** Calories: 220 kcal | Fat: 9 g | Protein: 4 g | Carbs: 31 g | Net carbs: 21 g | Fiber: 10 g | Cholesterol: 18 mg | Sodium: 960 mg | Potassium: 900 mg

**Useful Tip:** To make the soup even creamier, you can add a splash of extra heavy cream or a dollop of Greek yogurt before serving.

# Spiced Carrot and Ginger Soup

Serving: 4 | Prep time: 10 minutes | Cook time: 30 minutes

Ingredients:

- 16 oz (450 g) carrots, peeled and chopped
- 1 onion, chopped
- 2 cloves garlic, minced
- 1-inch (2.5 cm) piece of fresh ginger, peeled and grated
- 32 oz (960 ml) vegetable broth
- 1 tsp ground cumin
- 1/2 tsp ground coriander
- 1/4 tsp cayenne pepper
- 2 tbsp olive oil
- Salt and pepper to taste
- 2 tbsp coconut milk (for garnish)
- Fresh cilantro leaves (for garnish)

Directions:

1. In a large pot, heat the olive oil over medium heat. Add the chopped onion and cook until translucent.
2. Stir in the minced garlic and grated ginger. Sauté for another minute until fragrant.
3. Add the chopped carrots, ground cumin, ground coriander, and cayenne pepper. Cook for 5 minutes, stirring occasionally.
4. Pour in the vegetable broth, season with salt and pepper, and bring to a boil. Reduce heat, cover, and simmer for 20-25 minutes or until the carrots are tender.
5. Use an immersion blender or countertop blender to purée the soup until smooth.
6. Serve the soup hot, garnished with a drizzle of coconut milk and fresh cilantro leaves.

**Nutritional Values:** Calories: 120 kcal | Fat: 5 g | Protein: 2 g | Carbs: 18 g | Net carbs: 11 g | Fiber: 7 g | Cholesterol: 0 mg | Sodium: 680 mg | Potassium: 500 mg

**Useful Tip:** For added depth of flavor, you can toast the ground cumin and coriander in the pot for about 1 minute before adding the carrots.

## Vegan Split Pea Soup with Smoked Paprika

Serving: 4 | Prep time: 10 minutes | Cook time: 40 minutes

Ingredients:

- 8 oz (225 g) green split peas
- 1 onion, chopped
- 2 carrots, peeled and diced
- 2 celery stalks, chopped
- 32 oz (960 ml) vegetable broth
- 1 tsp smoked paprika
- 2 cloves garlic, minced
- 2 tbsp olive oil
- Salt and pepper to taste

Directions:

1. In a large pot, heat 1 tablespoon of olive oil over medium heat. Add the chopped onion, carrots, and celery. Sauté for about 5 minutes or until the vegetables are tender.
2. Rinse the green split peas and add them to the pot. Pour in the vegetable broth and bring to a boil. Reduce heat, cover, and simmer for 30-35 minutes or until the peas are soft.
3. Using an immersion blender or countertop blender, purée the soup until smooth.
4. Return the soup to the pot, stir in the smoked paprika and minced garlic. Season with salt and pepper. Heat the soup over low heat until it's warm.

**Nutritional Values:** Calories: 180 kcal | Fat: 6 g | Protein: 6 g | Carbs: 28 g | Net carbs: 19 g | Fiber: 9 g | Cholesterol: 0 mg | Sodium: 680 mg | Potassium: 570 mg

**Useful Tip:** Add a dollop of vegan sour cream and a sprinkle of fresh chopped chives for extra flavor.

# Roasted Red Pepper and Chickpea Soup

Serving: 4 | Prep time: 15 minutes | Cook time: 30 minutes

Ingredients:

- 2 large red bell peppers
- 1 can (15 oz / 425 g) chickpeas, drained and rinsed
- 1 onion, chopped
- 2 cloves garlic, minced
- 32 oz (960 ml) vegetable broth
- 2 tbsp olive oil
- 1 tsp cumin
- 1/2 tsp paprika
- Salt and pepper to taste
- Fresh cilantro leaves for garnish

Directions:

1. Preheat your oven to 450°F (230°C). Place the whole red bell peppers on a baking sheet and roast for about 25-30 minutes, turning occasionally until the skin is charred and blistered.
2. Remove the roasted bell peppers from the oven and place them in a bowl covered with plastic wrap. Let them steam for about 10 minutes; this will make it easier to peel the skin.
3. Once the bell peppers are cool enough to handle, peel off the skin, remove the seeds, and chop them into small pieces.
4. In a large pot, heat the olive oil over medium heat. Add the chopped onion and cook until it becomes translucent.
5. Stir in the minced garlic, cumin, and paprika. Cook for another 1-2 minutes until fragrant.
6. Add the roasted red peppers, chickpeas, and vegetable broth to the pot. Season with salt and pepper. Bring the mixture to a boil, then reduce the heat and let it simmer for 10-15 minutes.
7. Use an immersion blender or countertop blender to purée the soup until it's smooth and creamy.
8. Serve the roasted red pepper and chickpea soup hot, garnished with fresh cilantro leaves.

**Nutritional Values:** Calories: 220 kcal | Fat: 8 g | Protein: 7 g | Carbs: 30 g | Net carbs: 20 g | Fiber: 10 g | Cholesterol: 0 mg | Sodium: 750 mg | Potassium: 580 mg

**Useful Tip:** For an extra flavor boost, drizzle some extra virgin olive oil over the soup just before serving.

# Mushroom and Barley Soup with Herbs

Serving: 4 | Prep time: 15 minutes | Cook time: 40 minutes

Ingredients:

- 8 oz (225 g) mushrooms, sliced
- 6 oz (180 g) barley
- 1 onion, finely chopped
- 2 cloves garlic, minced
- 32 oz (960 ml) vegetable broth
- 2 tbsp olive oil
- 1 tsp dried thyme
- 1 tsp dried rosemary
- Salt and pepper to taste
- Fresh parsley for garnish

Directions:

1. In a large pot, heat the olive oil over medium heat. Add the chopped onion and cook until it becomes translucent.

2. Stir in the minced garlic, dried thyme, and dried rosemary. Cook for another 1-2 minutes until fragrant.
3. Add the sliced mushrooms and barley to the pot. Cook for about 5 minutes, stirring occasionally.
4. Pour in the vegetable broth and bring the mixture to a boil.
5. Reduce the heat to a simmer, cover the pot, and let it cook for 30-35 minutes, or until the barley is tender.
6. Season the soup with salt and pepper to taste.
7. Serve the mushroom and barley soup hot, garnished with fresh parsley.

**Nutritional Values:** Calories: 320 kcal | Fat: 7 g | Protein: 7 g | Carbs: 60 g | Net carbs: 50 g | Fiber: 10 g | Cholesterol: 0 mg | Sodium: 780 mg | Potassium: 480 mg

**Useful Tip:** For an extra burst of flavor, squeeze a little fresh lemon juice into your bowl just before eating.

# SMOOTHIES

## Tropical Sunrise Smoothie

Serving: 4 | Prep time: 10 minutes | Cook time: 0 minutes

Ingredients:

- 8 oz (225 g) frozen mango chunks
- 8 oz (225 g) frozen pineapple chunks
- 4 oz (120 ml) coconut milk
- 4 oz (120 ml) orange juice
- 1 ripe banana
- 1 tsp honey (optional)
- 4 oz (120 ml) water
- Ice cubes
- Fresh mint leaves for garnish

Directions:

1. In a blender, combine the frozen mango chunks, frozen pineapple chunks, coconut milk, orange juice, ripe banana, and honey (if desired).
2. Add the water and a handful of ice cubes for an extra chill.
3. Blend all the ingredients until smooth and creamy. If the consistency is too thick, add more water as needed.
4. Pour the tropical sunrise smoothie into glasses.
5. Garnish each glass with a fresh mint leaf for a burst of freshness.

**Nutritional Values:** Calories: 180 kcal | Fat: 3 g | Protein: 2 g | Carbs: 41 g | Net carbs: 33 g | Fiber: 5 g | Cholesterol: 0 mg | Sodium: 5 mg | Potassium: 410 mg

**Useful Tip:** Customize your smoothie by adding a scoop of protein powder for an extra protein boost.

## Berry Blast Smoothie

Serving: 4 | Prep time: 5 minutes | Cook time: 0 minutes

Ingredients:

- 10 oz (280 g) frozen mixed berries (strawberries, blueberries, raspberries, and blackberries)
- 6 oz (180 ml) Greek yogurt
- 4 oz (120 ml) almond milk
- 2 oz (60 g) honey or to taste
- 1 ripe banana
- 4 oz (120 ml) water
- Ice cubes
- Fresh mint leaves for garnish

Directions:

1. In a blender, combine the frozen mixed berries, Greek yogurt, almond milk, honey, and a ripe banana.
2. Add the water and a handful of ice cubes for a refreshing chill.
3. Blend all the ingredients until the smoothie is thick and luscious. Adjust sweetness by adding more honey if desired.
4. Pour the Berry Blast Smoothie into glasses.
5. Garnish each glass with fresh mint leaves for a delightful touch.

Nutritional Values: Calories: 180 kcal | Fat: 1 g | Protein: 6 g | Carbs: 42 g | Net carbs: 35 g | Fiber: 7 g | Cholesterol: 2 mg | Sodium: 30 mg | Potassium: 300 mg

Useful Tip: For an extra protein boost, you can add a scoop of protein powder to your smoothie.

## Green Energy Smoothie

Serving: 4 | Prep time: 5 minutes | Cook time: 0 minutes

Ingredients:

- 6 oz (170 g) fresh spinach leaves
- 2 ripe avocados, peeled and pitted
- 2 oz (60 g) cucumber, peeled and chopped
- 4 oz (120 ml) coconut water
- 4 oz (120 ml) almond milk
- 2 oz (60 g) fresh pineapple chunks
- 1 oz (30 g) fresh mint leaves
- Juice of 1 lime
- Honey or agave nectar, to taste
- Ice cubes

Directions:

1. In a blender, combine the fresh spinach, ripe avocados, cucumber, coconut water, almond milk, fresh pineapple chunks, mint leaves, and lime juice.
2. Add honey or agave nectar to sweeten according to your taste.
3. Toss in a few ice cubes to make your smoothie refreshing.
4. Blend all the ingredients until your Green Energy Smoothie is silky smooth and vibrantly green.
5. Pour into glasses and garnish with additional mint leaves.

Nutritional Values: Calories: 150 kcal | Fat: 9 g | Protein: 2 g | Carbs: 19 g | Net carbs: 10 g | Fiber: 9 g | Cholesterol: 0 mg | Sodium: 80 mg | Potassium: 610 mg

Useful Tip: To enhance the protein content, you can add a scoop of your favorite protein powder or Greek yogurt.

## Citrus Splash Smoothie

Serving: 4 | Prep time: 5 minutes | Cook time: 0 minutes

Ingredients:

- 6 oz (170 g) Greek yogurt
- 2 oranges, peeled and segmented
- 1 grapefruit, peeled and segmented
- 2 oz (60 ml) fresh lime juice
- 2 oz (60 ml) honey
- 1 tbsp chia seeds
- Ice cubes

Directions:

1. In a blender, combine the Greek yogurt, segmented oranges, segmented grapefruit, fresh lime juice, and honey.
2. Add chia seeds to the mixture for an extra health boost.
3. Toss in a handful of ice cubes for a refreshing chill.
4. Blend all the ingredients until your Citrus Splash Smoothie is smooth and creamy.
5. Pour into glasses and garnish with additional citrus segments.

**Useful Tip:** Adjust the honey to your desired sweetness level and consider adding a few fresh mint leaves for an extra burst of flavor.

## Creamy Avocado Delight

Serving: 4 | Prep time: 10 minutes | Cook time: 0 minutes

### Ingredients:

- 2 ripe avocados, peeled and pitted (approximately 10 oz / 280 g each)
- 8 oz (230 g) Greek yogurt
- 4 oz (120 ml) unsweetened almond milk
- 1 lime, juiced and zested
- 1 oz (30 g) fresh cilantro leaves
- 1/2 tsp hot sauce
- Salt and pepper to taste

### Directions:

1. In a food processor or blender, combine the ripe avocados, Greek yogurt, unsweetened almond milk, lime juice, and lime zest.
2. Add fresh cilantro leaves and a touch of hot sauce for some zesty heat.
3. Season with salt and pepper to your taste preferences.
4. Blend until the mixture is smooth and creamy.
5. Chill the Creamy Avocado Delight in the refrigerator before serving for a refreshing taste.

**Nutritional Values:** Calories: 195 kcal | Fat: 14 g | Protein: 7 g | Carbs: 14 g | Net carbs: 6 g | Fiber: 8 g | Cholesterol: 3 mg | Sodium: 68 mg | Potassium: 642 mg

**Useful Tip:** Customize the hot sauce level to suit your spice preference, and consider adding a dollop of Greek yogurt or a sprinkle of toasted pumpkin seeds as a garnish.

## Mango Tango Smoothie

Serving: 4 | Prep time: 5 minutes | Cook time: 0 minutes

### Ingredients:

- 16 oz (450 g) frozen mango chunks
- 8 oz (240 ml) unsweetened coconut milk
- 8 oz (240 ml) orange juice
- 2 oz (60 g) Greek yogurt
- 1 tbsp honey
- 1 tsp vanilla extract
- 1/2 tsp ground turmeric
- Ice cubes (optional)

### Directions:

1. In a blender, combine the frozen mango chunks, unsweetened coconut milk, and orange juice.
2. Add Greek yogurt, honey, vanilla extract, and a touch of ground turmeric for extra vibrancy.
3. If you prefer a colder smoothie, feel free to add a handful of ice cubes.
4. Blend until the mixture is smooth and the desired consistency is reached.
5. Pour into glasses and garnish with a slice of fresh mango or a sprinkle of shredded coconut.

**Nutritional Values:** Calories: 185 kcal | Fat: 3 g | Protein: 3 g | Carbs: 42 g | Net carbs: 36 g | Fiber: 6 g | Cholesterol: 2 mg | Sodium: 42 mg | Potassium: 515 mg

**Useful Tip:** Turmeric adds a mild earthy flavor and a burst of color to this smoothie. Adjust the honey to meet your preferred sweetness level.

## Pomegranate Paradise

Serving: 4 | Prep time: 10 minutes | Cook time: 0 minutes

**Ingredients:**

- 16 oz (450 g) pomegranate seeds (approximately 2 pomegranates)
- 8 oz (240 ml) coconut water
- 8 oz (240 ml) plain Greek yogurt
- 2 tbsp honey
- 1 tsp lime juice
- 1/2 tsp vanilla extract
- Ice cubes (optional)

**Directions:**

1. Extract the seeds from the pomegranates (or you can use pre-packaged pomegranate seeds).
2. In a blender, combine the pomegranate seeds, coconut water, and plain Greek yogurt.
3. Add honey, lime juice, and a hint of vanilla extract to enhance the flavors.
4. If you like your smoothie chilled, toss in a few ice cubes.
5. Blend until you achieve a smooth consistency.
6. Pour into glasses and garnish with a sprinkle of pomegranate seeds or a lime wheel.

**Nutritional Values:** Calories: 178 kcal | Fat: 2 g | Protein: 9 g | Carbs: 33 g | Net carbs: 27 g | Fiber: 6 g | Cholesterol: 3 mg | Sodium: 73 mg | Potassium: 446 mg

**Useful Tip:** To easily extract pomegranate seeds, cut the fruit in half, hold it over a bowl cut side down, and tap the back with a wooden spoon.

## Papaya Passion Smoothie

Serving: 4 | Prep time: 10 minutes | Cook time: 0 minutes

**Ingredients:**

- 16 oz (450 g) ripe papaya, peeled, seeded, and cubed
- 8 oz (240 ml) orange juice
- 8 oz (240 ml) unsweetened almond milk
- 2 tbsp honey
- 1/2 tsp fresh lime juice
- 4 oz (120 g) plain Greek yogurt
- Ice cubes (optional)

**Directions:**

1. Prepare the papaya by peeling, removing seeds, and cutting into cubes.
2. In a blender, combine the papaya cubes, orange juice, unsweetened almond milk, honey, lime juice, and plain Greek yogurt.
3. Add ice cubes if you prefer your smoothie extra cold.
4. Blend until the mixture is smooth and creamy.
5. Pour into glasses, garnish with a papaya slice or a twist of lime, and serve.

**Nutritional Values:** Calories: 128 kcal | Fat: 1 g | Protein: 5 g | Carbs: 27 g | Net carbs: 24 g | Fiber: 3 g | Cholesterol: 2 mg | Sodium: 72 mg | Potassium: 332 mg

**Useful Tip:** To easily cube the papaya, cut it in half lengthwise, scoop out the seeds, and use a spoon to separate the flesh from the skin. Then, chop it into small pieces.

## Banana and Almond Bliss

Serving: 4 | Prep time: 5 minutes | Cook time: 0 minutes

**Ingredients:**

- 4 ripe bananas, peeled and sliced
- 12 oz (340 g) unsweetened almond milk
- 2 oz (60 g) almond butter
- 2 tbsp honey
- 1/2 tsp pure vanilla extract
- 1/2 tsp ground cinnamon
- Ice cubes (optional)

**Directions:**

1. Peel and slice the ripe bananas.
2. In a blender, combine the banana slices, unsweetened almond milk, almond butter, honey, pure vanilla extract, and ground cinnamon.
3. Add ice cubes if you prefer your smoothie extra cold.
4. Blend until the mixture is smooth and creamy.
5. Pour into glasses, garnish with a sprinkle of ground cinnamon or a banana slice, and serve.

**Nutritional Values:** Calories: 232 kcal | Fat: 9 g | Protein: 4 g | Carbs: 36 g | Net carbs: 27 g | Fiber: 9 g | Cholesterol: 0 mg | Sodium: 93 mg | Potassium: 485 mg

**Useful Tip:** For a thicker smoothie, freeze the banana slices before blending, or use a frozen banana.

## Spinach and Pineapple Pleasure

Serving: 4 | Prep time: 5 minutes | Cook time: 0 minutes

**Ingredients:**

- 6 oz (170 g) fresh spinach leaves
- 16 oz (480 ml) unsweetened pineapple juice
- 16 oz (480 ml) coconut water
- 8 oz (240 ml) plain Greek yogurt
- 2 tablespoons honey
- 8 oz (240 ml) ice cubes
- Fresh pineapple chunks for garnish (optional)

**Directions:**

1. Place the fresh spinach leaves in a blender.
2. Add unsweetened pineapple juice, coconut water, plain Greek yogurt, and honey.
3. Top with a cup of ice cubes.
4. Blend until the mixture is smooth and the spinach is completely incorporated.
5. Pour into glasses, garnish with fresh pineapple chunks if desired, and serve.

**Nutritional Values:** Calories: 131 kcal | Fat: 1 g | Protein: 5 g | Carbs: 30 g | Net carbs: 25 g | Fiber: 5 g | Cholesterol: 1 mg | Sodium: 94 mg | Potassium: 689 mg

# HOMEMADE PROTEIN SHAKES

## Vanilla Almond Protein Shake

Serving: 4 | Prep Time: 5 minutes | Cook Time: 0 minutes

**Ingredients:**

- 8 oz (240 g) almond milk
- 12 oz (360 g) Greek yogurt
- 4 oz (120 g) vanilla protein powder
- 2 oz (60 g) almond butter
- 1 oz (30 g) honey
- 1 tsp vanilla extract
- 1/2 tsp ground cinnamon
- 8 ice cubes

**Directions:**

1. In a blender, combine the almond milk, Greek yogurt, vanilla protein powder, almond butter, honey, vanilla extract, and ground cinnamon.
2. Add the ice cubes to the blender.
3. Blend all the ingredients on high until the shake is smooth and creamy.
4. Pour the Vanilla Almond Protein Shake into four glasses.
5. Optionally, sprinkle a pinch of cinnamon on top for garnish.
6. Serve immediately and enjoy the refreshing taste!

**Nutritional Values:** Calories: 220 kcal | Fat: 8 g | Protein: 23 g | Carbs: 15 g | Net Carbs: 14 g | Fiber: 1 g | Cholesterol: 30 mg | Sodium: 120 mg | Potassium: 250 mg

**Useful Tip:** You can adjust the sweetness by adding more or less honey based on your personal preference.

## Chocolate Peanut Butter Power Shake

Serving: 4 | Prep Time: 5 minutes | Cook Time: 0 minutes

**Ingredients:**

- 8 oz (240 g) almond milk
- 4 oz (120 g) chocolate protein powder
- 2 oz (60 g) peanut butter
- 1 oz (30 g) honey
- 1/2 oz (15 g) cocoa powder
- 1 tsp vanilla extract
- 6 ice cubes
- 2 tbsp Greek yogurt

**Directions:**

1. In a blender, add the almond milk, chocolate protein powder, peanut butter, honey, cocoa powder, and vanilla extract.
2. Drop in the ice cubes and Greek yogurt.
3. Blend on high until the shake is smooth and all ingredients are well combined.
4. Pour the Chocolate Peanut Butter Power Shake into four glasses.
5. Optionally, drizzle some extra honey on top as a sweet garnish.
6. Serve immediately and savor the rich, chocolatey goodness!

Nutritional Values: Calories: 280 kcal | Fat: 9 g | Protein: 24 g | Carbs: 22 g | Net Carbs: 19 g | Fiber: 3 g | Cholesterol: 15 mg | Sodium: 180 mg | Potassium: 280 mg

Useful Tip: If you prefer a thicker consistency, add more ice cubes or Greek yogurt. Adjust the sweetness by adding extra honey if desired.

## Blueberry Blast Protein Shake

Serving: 4 | Prep Time: 5 minutes | Cook Time: 0 minutes

Ingredients:

- 10 oz (300 g) almond milk
- 4 oz (120 g) blueberries (fresh or frozen)
- 4 oz (120 g) vanilla protein powder
- 2 oz (60 g) Greek yogurt
- 1 oz (30 g) honey
- 1 tsp lemon zest
- 6 ice cubes

Directions:

1. In a blender, add the almond milk, blueberries, vanilla protein powder, Greek yogurt, honey, and lemon zest.
2. Drop in the ice cubes to help chill and thicken the shake.
3. Blend on high until the shake is smooth and the blueberries are fully incorporated.
4. Pour the Blueberry Blast Protein Shake into four glasses.
5. For added freshness, garnish with a few extra blueberries or a sprinkle of lemon zest.
6. Serve immediately and enjoy the refreshing burst of blueberry flavor!

Nutritional Values: Calories: 240 kcal | Fat: 4 g | Protein: 24 g | Carbs: 27 g | Net Carbs: 23 g | Fiber: 4 g | Cholesterol: 10 mg | Sodium: 150 mg | Potassium: 310 mg

Useful Tip: To make it even creamier, you can substitute almond milk with coconut milk or regular milk. Adjust the sweetness by adding more or less honey according to your taste.

## Coconut Macaroon Muscle Shake

Serving: 4 | Prep Time: 5 minutes | Cook Time: 0 minutes

Ingredients:

- 10 oz (300 g) coconut milk
- 4 oz (120 g) shredded coconut
- 4 oz (120 g) vanilla protein powder
- 2 oz (60 g) almond butter
- 1 oz (30 g) honey
- 1 tsp coconut extract
- 6 ice cubes
- 2 tbsp Greek yogurt

Directions:

1. In a blender, combine the coconut milk, shredded coconut, vanilla protein powder, almond butter, honey, and coconut extract.
2. Add the ice cubes and Greek yogurt to the blender for a creamy texture.
3. Blend on high until all the ingredients are well combined and the shake is smooth.
4. Pour the Coconut Macaroon Muscle Shake into four glasses.
5. Optionally, sprinkle some additional shredded coconut on top for extra crunch.

6. Serve immediately and savor the tropical coconut goodness!

**Nutritional Values:** Calories: 280 kcal | Fat: 15 g | Protein: 22 g | Carbs: 20 g | Net Carbs: 15 g | Fiber: 5 g | Cholesterol: 10 mg | Sodium: 130 mg | Potassium: 320 mg

**Useful Tip:** For an extra protein boost, you can add a scoop of collagen powder or your favorite protein supplement without altering the flavor significantly.

## Mocha Espresso Protein Shake

Serving: 4 | Prep Time: 5 minutes | Cook Time: 0 minutes

**Ingredients:**

- 10 oz (300 g) brewed espresso, chilled
- 4 oz (120 g) chocolate protein powder
- 2 oz (60 g) almond butter
- 1 oz (30 g) honey
- 1 tsp cocoa powder
- 1/2 tsp instant coffee granules
- 8 ice cubes
- 2 tbsp Greek yogurt

**Directions:**

1. Start with chilled brewed espresso and add it to the blender.
2. Incorporate the chocolate protein powder, almond butter, honey, cocoa powder, and instant coffee granules.
3. Add the ice cubes and Greek yogurt for thickness and creaminess.
4. Blend on high until the shake is well mixed and has a velvety consistency.
5. Pour the Mocha Espresso Protein Shake into four glasses.
6. Optionally, dust with a sprinkle of cocoa powder for an extra mocha touch.
7. Serve immediately and enjoy your energizing and indulgent shake!

**Nutritional Values:** Calories: 280 kcal | Fat: 9 g | Protein: 24 g | Carbs: 23 g | Net Carbs: 18 g | Fiber: 5 g | Cholesterol: 10 mg | Sodium: 150 mg | Potassium: 280 mg

**Useful Tip:** To adjust the sweetness, add more or less honey, or use flavored Greek yogurt for an extra layer of taste.

## Strawberry Cheesecake Protein Shake

Serving: 4 | Prep Time: 5 minutes | Cook Time: 0 minutes

**Ingredients:**

- 8 oz (240 g) almond milk
- 4 oz (120 g) fresh or frozen strawberries
- 4 oz (120 g) vanilla protein powder
- 2 oz (60 g) cream cheese
- 1 oz (30 g) honey
- 1/2 tsp lemon zest
- 8 ice cubes
- 2 tbsp Greek yogurt

**Directions:**

1. In a blender, combine the almond milk, strawberries, vanilla protein powder, cream cheese, honey, and lemon zest.
2. Add the ice cubes and Greek yogurt to enhance the creaminess and coldness of the shake.
3. Blend on high until all the ingredients are thoroughly mixed and the shake is smooth.

4.  Pour the Strawberry Cheesecake Protein Shake into four glasses.

5.  Optionally, garnish with a strawberry slice or a sprinkle of lemon zest for an elegant touch.

6.  Serve immediately and savor the delightful taste reminiscent of strawberry cheesecake!

**Nutritional Values:** Calories: 270 kcal | Fat: 9 g | Protein: 24 g | Carbs: 20 g | Net Carbs: 18 g | Fiber: 2 g | Cholesterol: 20 mg | Sodium: 160 mg | Potassium: 280 mg

**Useful Tip:** To make it extra rich and creamy, you can substitute Greek yogurt with a small portion of cottage cheese or ricotta cheese.

## Banana Nut Protein Shake

Serving: 4 | Prep Time: 5 minutes | Cook Time: 0 minutes

**Ingredients:**

- 8 oz (240 g) almond milk
- 4 oz (120 g) ripe banana
- 4 oz (120 g) vanilla protein powder
- 2 oz (60 g) natural peanut butter
- 1 oz (30 g) honey
- 1/2 tsp cinnamon
- 8 ice cubes
- 2 tbsp chopped walnuts

**Directions:**

1.  In a blender, combine the almond milk, ripe banana, vanilla protein powder, natural peanut butter, honey, and a dash of cinnamon.

2.  Add the ice cubes to create a chilled and creamy shake.

3.  Blend on high until all ingredients are well combined and the shake is smooth.

4.  Pour the Banana Nut Protein Shake into four glasses.

5.  Top each serving with chopped walnuts for a delightful crunch.

6.  Serve immediately and enjoy the delicious blend of banana and nut flavors!

**Nutritional Values:** Calories: 280 kcal | Fat: 9 g | Protein: 24 g | Carbs: 22 g | Net Carbs: 18 g | Fiber: 4 g | Cholesterol: 10 mg | Sodium: 140 mg | Potassium: 300 mg

**Useful Tip:** You can adjust the thickness by adding more ice cubes or almond milk as needed, and for extra protein, try adding a scoop of powdered collagen or a protein supplement of your choice.

## Mixed Berry Protein Refuel

Serving: 4 | Prep Time: 5 minutes | Cook Time: 0 minutes

**Ingredients:**

- 8 oz (240 g) unsweetened almond milk
- 4 oz (120 g) mixed berries (strawberries, blueberries, and raspberries)
- 4 oz (120 g) vanilla protein powder
- 2 oz (60 g) plain Greek yogurt
- 1 oz (30 g) honey
- 1/2 tsp lemon juice
- 8 ice cubes
- 1 tbsp chia seeds

**Directions:**

1.  In a blender, combine unsweetened almond milk, mixed berries, vanilla protein powder, plain Greek yogurt, honey, and a squeeze of lemon juice.
2.  Add the ice cubes to give your shake a refreshing chill and thickness.
3.  Blend until all ingredients are well combined, and the texture is smooth.
4.  Pour the Mixed Berry Protein Refuel into four glasses.
5.  Sprinkle chia seeds on top for added texture and a boost of healthy omega-3 fatty acids.
6.  Serve immediately and enjoy the vibrant and nutritious flavors!

**Nutritional Values:** Calories: 280 kcal | Fat: 8 g | Protein: 24 g | Carbs: 27 g | Net Carbs: 18 g | Fiber: 9 g | Cholesterol: 10 mg | Sodium: 120 mg | Potassium: 260 mg

**Useful Tip:** Chia seeds not only add a delightful crunch but also provide a healthy dose of fiber, making this shake more filling and satisfying.

# Cookies and Cream Protein Shake

Serving: 4 | Prep Time: 5 minutes | Cook Time: 0 minutes

**Ingredients:**

- 8 oz (240 g) unsweetened almond milk
- 4 oz (120 g) chocolate protein powder
- 2 oz (60 g) reduced-fat cream cheese
- 1 oz (30 g) dark chocolate cookies (crushed)
- 1 oz (30 g) honey
- 1/2 tsp vanilla extract
- 8 ice cubes
- 2 tbsp whipped cream

**Directions:**

1.  In a blender, combine unsweetened almond milk, chocolate protein powder, reduced-fat cream cheese, crushed dark chocolate cookies, honey, and a dash of vanilla extract.
2.  Add ice cubes for thickness and a delightful chill to your shake.
3.  Blend until all ingredients are thoroughly combined, and the shake is smooth.
4.  Pour the Cookies and Cream Protein Shake into four glasses.
5.  Top each serving with a dollop of whipped cream for a decadent touch.
6.  Serve immediately and relish the indulgent cookies and cream goodness!

**Nutritional Values:** Calories: 280 kcal | Fat: 10 g | Protein: 25 g | Carbs: 21 g | Net Carbs: 18 g | Fiber: 3 g | Cholesterol: 20 mg | Sodium: 150 mg | Potassium: 280 mg

**Useful Tip:** Adjust the sweetness to your liking by adding more or less honey, and for an extra protein boost, incorporate a scoop of your favorite protein supplement.

# Pumpkin Spice Protein Shake

Serving: 4 | Prep Time: 5 minutes | Cook Time: 0 minutes

## Ingredients:

- 8 oz (240 g) unsweetened almond milk
- 4 oz (120 g) canned pumpkin puree
- 4 oz (120 g) vanilla protein powder
- 2 oz (60 g) plain Greek yogurt
- 1 oz (30 g) honey
- 1/2 tsp pumpkin spice mix
- 8 ice cubes
- 2 tbsp whipped cream (optional)

## Directions:

1. In a blender, combine unsweetened almond milk, canned pumpkin puree, vanilla protein powder, plain Greek yogurt, honey, and a sprinkle of pumpkin spice mix.
2. Add ice cubes to create a creamy and chilled texture.
3. Blend until all ingredients are well combined, and the shake is smooth.
4. Pour the Pumpkin Spice Protein Shake into four glasses.
5. Optionally, top each serving with a dollop of whipped cream for an extra layer of decadence.
6. Serve immediately and delight in the cozy pumpkin spice flavors!

**Nutritional Values:** Calories: 260 kcal | Fat: 7 g | Protein: 25 g | Carbs: 23 g | Net Carbs: 16 g | Fiber: 7 g | Cholesterol: 15 mg | Sodium: 160 mg | Potassium: 260 mg

**Useful Tip:** For an even richer pumpkin flavor, roast fresh pumpkin slices in the oven and puree them as a substitute for canned pumpkin puree.

# DESSERTS

## Cacao and Almond Protein Bars

Serving: 4 | Prep Time: 15 minutes | Cook Time: 0 minutes

Ingredients:

- 6 oz (180 g) rolled oats
- 4 oz (120 g) almond butter
- 2 oz (60 g) cacao powder
- 2 oz (60 g) honey
- 1 oz (30 g) almond slices
- 1 tsp vanilla extract
- 1/2 tsp sea salt
- 4 oz (120 ml) unsweetened almond milk

Directions:

1. In a large mixing bowl, combine rolled oats, almond butter, cacao powder, honey, almond slices, vanilla extract, and a pinch of sea salt.
2. Gradually add unsweetened almond milk while stirring until the mixture reaches a dough-like consistency.
3. Press the mixture into a square or rectangular baking dish lined with parchment paper, ensuring it's evenly spread and compact.
4. Place the dish in the refrigerator for at least 2 hours to set.
5. Once firm, remove the mixture from the dish and cut it into bars or squares.
6. Store the Cacao and Almond Protein Bars in an airtight container in the fridge for a quick and nutritious snack.

Nutritional Values: Calories: 280 kcal | Fat: 15 g | Protein: 8 g | Carbs: 32 g | Net Carbs: 25 g | Fiber: 7 g | Cholesterol: 0 mg | Sodium: 120 mg | Potassium: 240 mg

Useful Tip: To enhance the flavor, you can add a handful of cacao nibs or dark chocolate chips to the mixture before refrigerating.

## Pumpkin Pie Protein Brownies

Serving: 4 | Prep Time: 15 minutes | Cook Time: 25 minutes

Ingredients:

- 4 oz (120 g) pumpkin puree
- 4 oz (120 g) chocolate protein powder
- 2 oz (60 g) almond butter
- 2 oz (60 g) honey
- 1 oz (30 g) cacao powder
- 1 tsp pumpkin pie spice
- 1/2 tsp baking soda
- 2 oz (60 ml) unsweetened almond milk

Directions:

1. Preheat your oven to 350°F (175°C) and line a square baking dish with parchment paper.
2. In a mixing bowl, combine pumpkin puree, chocolate protein powder, almond butter, honey, cacao powder, pumpkin pie spice, and baking soda.
3. Add unsweetened almond milk and mix until the batter is smooth and well incorporated.
4. Pour the batter into the prepared baking dish, spreading it evenly.

5. Bake for approximately 25 minutes or until a toothpick comes out clean.

6. Let the brownies cool in the dish for a few minutes, then transfer them to a wire rack to cool completely.

7. Once cooled, cut the Pumpkin Pie Protein Brownies into squares and enjoy your guilt-free treat!

**Nutritional Values:** Calories: 220 kcal | Fat: 10 g | Protein: 15 g | Carbs: 20 g | Net Carbs: 15 g | Fiber: 5 g | Cholesterol: 5 mg | Sodium: 180 mg | Potassium: 250 mg

**Useful Tip:** For extra indulgence, you can drizzle melted dark chocolate or sprinkle chopped nuts on top before the brownies set.

# Lemon Poppy Seed Protein Pancakes

Serving: 4 | Prep Time: 10 minutes | Cook Time: 15 minutes

## Ingredients:

- 4 oz (120 g) oat flour
- 4 oz (120 g) lemon-flavored protein powder
- 2 oz (60 g) Greek yogurt
- 1 oz (30 g) almond milk
- 2 oz (60 g) egg whites
- 1 oz (30 g) lemon juice
- 1/2 oz (15 g) honey
- 1 tsp poppy seeds
- 1/2 tsp baking powder
- Zest of 1 lemon
- Cooking spray (for the pan)

## Directions:

1. In a mixing bowl, combine oat flour, lemon-flavored protein powder, Greek yogurt, almond milk, egg whites, lemon juice, honey, poppy seeds, baking powder, and lemon zest.

2. Mix until the batter is smooth and well blended.

3. Heat a non-stick skillet over medium heat and lightly coat it with cooking spray.

4. Pour 1/4 cup of the batter onto the skillet for each pancake.

5. Cook for about 2-3 minutes on each side, or until bubbles form on the surface and the edges are set.

6. Flip the pancakes and cook for another 2-3 minutes until they are golden brown and cooked through.

7. Serve the Lemon Poppy Seed Protein Pancakes hot, garnished with extra lemon zest and a drizzle of honey.

**Nutritional Values:** Calories: 280 kcal | Fat: 5 g | Protein: 25 g | Carbs: 35 g | Net Carbs: 30 g | Fiber: 5 g | Cholesterol: 15 mg | Sodium: 220 mg | Potassium: 280 mg

**Useful Tip:** If the batter is too thick, you can adjust the consistency by adding a bit more almond milk until you reach the desired thickness for your pancakes.

# Carrot Cake Protein Cookies

Serving: 4 | Prep Time: 15 minutes | Cook Time: 12 minutes

## Ingredients:

- 4 oz (120 g) rolled oats
- 4 oz (120 g) vanilla protein powder
- 2 oz (60 g) shredded carrots
- 1 oz (30 g) unsweetened applesauce
- 1 oz (30 g) honey
- 1/2 oz (15 g) chopped walnuts
- 1/2 tsp ground cinnamon
- 1/4 tsp ground nutmeg

- 1/4 tsp baking powder
- 1/4 tsp salt

**Directions:**

1. Preheat your oven to 350°F (175°C) and line a baking sheet with parchment paper.
2. In a food processor, blend rolled oats until they reach a flour-like consistency.
3. In a mixing bowl, combine oat flour, vanilla protein powder, shredded carrots, unsweetened applesauce, honey, chopped walnuts, ground cinnamon, ground nutmeg, baking powder, and salt.
4. Mix until all the ingredients form a thick cookie dough.
5. Form the dough into 12 equal portions, shape them into cookies, and place them on the prepared baking sheet.
6. Bake for approximately 12 minutes or until the cookies are firm and lightly golden.
7. Let the Carrot Cake Protein Cookies cool on a wire rack before serving.

**Nutritional Values:** Calories: 220 kcal | Fat: 8 g | Protein: 15 g | Carbs: 24 g | Net Carbs: 18 g | Fiber: 6 g | Cholesterol: 5 mg | Sodium: 160 mg | Potassium: 240 mg

**Useful Tip:** If your protein powder is unsweetened, you can adjust the sweetness by adding a bit more honey or a touch of your favorite sweetener to the dough.

# Orange Zest Madeleines

Serving: 4 | Prep Time: 15 minutes | Cook Time: 12 minutes

**Ingredients:**

- 4 oz (120 g) all-purpose flour
- 2 oz (60 g) unsalted butter, melted and cooled
- 2 oz (60 g) granulated sugar
- 1 oz (30 g) almond meal
- 1 oz (30 g) orange zest
- 1/2 oz (15 g) honey
- 1/2 oz (15 g) fresh orange juice
- 1/2 tsp baking powder
- 2 large eggs
- Pinch of salt

**Directions:**

1. Preheat your oven to 350°F (175°C) and grease a madeleine pan with a little melted butter.
2. In a mixing bowl, whisk together all-purpose flour, almond meal, baking powder, and a pinch of salt.
3. In another bowl, whisk together eggs and granulated sugar until light and creamy.
4. Add melted butter, honey, fresh orange juice, and orange zest to the egg mixture. Mix until well combined.
5. Gradually fold the dry ingredients into the wet ingredients until a smooth batter forms.
6. Spoon the batter into the prepared madeleine pan, filling each mold about two-thirds full.
7. Bake for 10-12 minutes or until the madeleines are golden around the edges and spring back when lightly touched.
8. Remove the madeleines from the pan and let them cool on a wire rack.

**Nutritional Values:** Calories: 200 kcal | Fat: 10 g | Protein: 4 g | Carbs: 25 g | Net Carbs: 20 g | Fiber: 5 g | Cholesterol: 65 mg | Sodium: 80 mg | Potassium: 150 mg

**Useful Tip:** To enhance the orange flavor, you can glaze the madeleines with a mixture of powdered sugar and orange juice once they have cooled completely.

# Oatmeal Raisin Cookies

Serving: 4 | Prep Time: 15 minutes | Cook Time: 12 minutes

Ingredients:

- 4 oz (120 g) rolled oats
- 2 oz (60 g) almond butter
- 2 oz (60 g) honey
- 2 oz (60 g) raisins
- 2 oz (60 g) unsweetened applesauce
- 1 oz (30 g) vanilla protein powder
- 1/2 oz (15 g) chopped walnuts
- 1/2 tsp ground cinnamon
- 1/4 tsp baking powder
- 1/4 tsp salt

Directions:

1. Preheat your oven to 350°F (175°C) and line a baking sheet with parchment paper.
2. In a mixing bowl, combine rolled oats, almond butter, honey, raisins, unsweetened applesauce, vanilla protein powder, chopped walnuts, ground cinnamon, baking powder, and salt.
3. Mix until all the ingredients form a thick cookie dough.
4. Form the dough into 12 equal portions, shape them into cookies, and place them on the prepared baking sheet.
5. Flatten each cookie slightly with the back of a spoon.
6. Bake for approximately 12 minutes or until the cookies are firm and lightly golden.
7. Let the Oatmeal Raisin Breakfast Cookies cool on a wire rack before serving.

Nutritional Values: Calories: 250 kcal | Fat: 9 g | Protein: 12 g | Carbs: 32 g | Net Carbs: 25 g | Fiber: 7 g | Cholesterol: 5 mg | Sodium: 160 mg | Potassium: 270 mg

Useful Tip: These cookies are perfect for a quick breakfast or snack on the go. You can customize them by adding your favorite nuts, seeds, or dried fruits.

# Gluten-Free Coconut Macaroons

Serving: 4 | Prep Time: 15 minutes | Cook Time: 20 minutes

Ingredients:

- 4 oz (120 g) shredded coconut
- 2 oz (60 g) honey
- 2 oz (60 g) egg whites (approximately 2 large eggs)
- 1 oz (30 g) almond flour
- 1 oz (30 g) coconut oil, melted
- 1 tsp vanilla extract
- 1/2 tsp salt
- 1/4 tsp almond extract (optional)

Directions:

1. Preheat your oven to 325°F (160°C) and line a baking sheet with parchment paper.
2. In a mixing bowl, combine shredded coconut, honey, egg whites, almond flour, melted coconut oil, vanilla extract, salt, and optional almond extract.
3. Mix until all the ingredients are well combined.
4. Using a cookie scoop or your hands, form the mixture into small mounds and place them on the prepared baking sheet.

5. Bake for 15-20 minutes or until the macaroons are lightly golden on the outside.
6. Remove from the oven and let them cool on the baking sheet for a few minutes.
7. Transfer the macaroons to a wire rack to cool completely.

**Nutritional Values:** Calories: 180 kcal | Fat: 10 g | Protein: 3 g | Carbs: 20 g | Net Carbs: 16 g | Fiber: 4 g | Cholesterol: 0 mg | Sodium: 250 mg | Potassium: 120 mg

**Useful Tip:** For an extra layer of flavor and a nice glossy finish, you can drizzle melted dark chocolate over the cooled macaroons.

# Greek Honey Nut Tartlets

Serving: 4 | Prep Time: 20 minutes | Cook Time: 20 minutes

## Ingredients:

- 4 oz (120 g) phyllo dough, thawed
- 2 oz (60 g) mixed nuts (walnuts, almonds, and pistachios), finely chopped
- 2 oz (60 g) honey
- 1 oz (30 g) unsalted butter, melted
- 1/2 oz (15 g) granulated sugar
- 1/2 tsp lemon juice
- 1/4 tsp ground cinnamon
- 1/8 tsp salt

## Directions:

1. Preheat your oven to 350°F (175°C).
2. In a bowl, combine the finely chopped mixed nuts, granulated sugar, ground cinnamon, and a pinch of salt. Mix well and set aside.
3. Place one sheet of phyllo dough on a clean surface and brush it with melted butter. Repeat with three more sheets, stacking them on top of each other and brushing each with butter.
4. Cut the layered phyllo sheets into 12 equal squares.
5. Place a spoonful of the nut mixture in the center of each square.
6. Gather the edges of each square and pinch them together to form a little pouch. Make sure they are sealed.
7. Place the tartlets on a baking sheet lined with parchment paper.
8. Bake in the preheated oven for about 15-20 minutes or until the tartlets are golden brown and crisp.
9. While still warm, drizzle honey over the tartlets, and then sprinkle them with a few drops of lemon juice.
10. Allow them to cool before serving.

**Nutritional Values:** Calories: 220 kcal | Fat: 12 g | Protein: 4 g | Carbs: 25 g | Net Carbs: 20 g | Fiber: 5 g | Cholesterol: 10 mg | Sodium: 190 mg | Potassium: 100 mg

**Useful Tip:** To ensure the phyllo dough doesn't dry out while working with it, cover the sheets you're not using with a damp kitchen towel.

# Pistachio and Apricot Rugelach

Serving: 4 | Prep Time: 25 minutes | Cook Time: 20 minutes

Ingredients:

- 8 oz (225 g) cream cheese, softened
- 4 oz (115 g) unsalted butter, softened
- 7 oz (200 g) all-purpose flour
- 1 oz (30 g) powdered sugar
- 2 oz (60 g) shelled pistachios, finely chopped
- 3 oz (85 g) dried apricots, finely chopped
- 2 tbsp honey
- 1/4 tsp salt

Directions:

1. In a large bowl, cream together the softened cream cheese and butter until smooth and creamy.
2. Gradually add the flour , salt and powdered sugar, mixing until the dough comes together.
3. Divide the dough into four equal portions, shape each portion into a disk, wrap in plastic wrap, and refrigerate for at least 1 hour.
4. Preheat your oven to 350°F (175°C) and line a baking sheet with parchment paper.
5. On a lightly floured surface, roll out one dough portion into a 1/8-inch thick circle.
6. Spread a thin layer of honey over the rolled-out dough, then sprinkle chopped pistachios and apricots evenly over the honey.
7. Using a sharp knife or a pizza cutter, cut the dough into 8 equal wedges.
8. Roll up each wedge from the wider end to form a crescent shape and place it on the prepared baking sheet.
9. Repeat steps 5-8 with the remaining dough portions.
10. Bake the rugelach in the preheated oven for 18-20 minutes or until golden brown.
11. Allow the rugelach to cool on the baking sheet for 5 minutes before transferring them to a wire rack to cool completely.

Nutritional Values: Calories: 380 kcal | Fat: 25 g | Protein: 6 g | Carbs: 35 g | Net Carbs: 30 g | Fiber: 5 g | Cholesterol: 65 mg | Sodium: 120 mg | Potassium: 250 mg

Useful Tip: To enhance the flavors, you can sprinkle a bit of cinnamon or cardamom along with the pistachios and apricots.

# Almond Biscotti with Dark Chocolate Drizzle

Serving: 4 | Prep Time: 20 minutes | Cook Time: 40 minutes

Ingredients:

- 7 oz (200 g) almond flour
- 2 oz (60 g) granulated sweetener (e.g., erythritol)
- 1 tsp baking powder
- 1/4 tsp salt
- 2 large eggs
- 1 tsp almond extract
- 2 oz (60 g) chopped roasted almonds
- 3 oz (85 g) sugar-free dark chocolate, melted

Directions:

1. Preheat your oven to 350°F (175°C) and line a baking sheet with parchment paper.
2. In a large mixing bowl, combine the almond flour, granulated sweetener, baking powder, and salt.

3. In a separate bowl, beat the eggs and almond extract together.
4. Pour the wet ingredients into the dry ingredients and mix until a dough forms.
5. Fold in the chopped roasted almonds.
6. Form the dough into a log shape on the prepared baking sheet.
7. Bake in the preheated oven for 25-30 minutes until the log is firm and lightly golden.
8. Remove the log from the oven and let it cool for 15 minutes.
9. Using a sharp knife, slice the log into 1/2-inch (1.25 cm) thick biscotti.
10. Place the biscotti back on the baking sheet and bake for an additional 10 minutes or until they're crisp and golden.
11. Allow the biscotti to cool completely.
12. Melt the sugar-free dark chocolate in a microwave or over a double boiler.
13. Drizzle the melted chocolate over the biscotti.
14. Let the chocolate set before serving.

**Nutritional Values:** Calories: 180 kcal | Fat: 15 g | Protein: 6 g | Carbs: 7 g | Net Carbs: 2 g | Fiber: 5 g | Cholesterol: 60 mg | Sodium: 230 mg | Potassium: 100 mg

**Useful Tip:** To make the drizzling process easier, you can pour the melted chocolate into a zip-top bag, cut a small hole in the corner, and use it to drizzle the chocolate over the biscotti.

# CONCLUSION

In closing, the Macro Cookbook for Beginners has been your compass through the intricacies of a macro-focused diet. This culinary journey has introduced you to the world of macronutrients, empowering you to create balanced, satisfying meals while working toward your unique dietary goals.

As you reach the end of this book, it's essential to reflect on the knowledge and skills you've gained. You've discovered the art of macro calculation, macro tracking flexibility, and nutrient balance importance. You've become adept at adapting your macros to meet your dietary preferences and restrictions, ensuring your culinary experience remains diverse and personalized.

Your kitchen has transformed into a hub of creativity and health, where you've explored recipes tailored to your macros, satisfying your taste buds and nutritional needs. You've navigated social gatherings and restaurant dining, applying your newfound macro wisdom to maintain consistency and control.

The glossary has given you a vocabulary that enhances your understanding of macros, enabling you to converse about nutrition with confidence and precision. You've armed yourself with helpful tools and resources that simplify your dietary journey, making it more accessible and enjoyable.

The FAQs and troubleshooting section has addressed common queries and challenges, offering guidance to help you overcome hurdles and maintain motivation. Your macro journey is uniquely yours, and with the knowledge and skills you've acquired from this book, you're well-prepared to continue your path to success.

Remember, the Macro Cookbook for Beginners is not merely a collection of recipes but a comprehensive guide to a sustainable, balanced way of eating. It equips you with the knowledge, tools, and inspiration to make informed choices, track your progress, and adapt to your evolving dietary needs.

As you continue your macro journey, embrace this diet's flexibility, creativity, and balance. Trust in the principles you've learned and the skills you've honed. Understanding macros will be your guiding light, whether your goal is weight management, muscle gain, or a healthier lifestyle.

It's time to start your culinary adventure, shaped by your unique tastes, preferences, and aspirations. The Macro Cookbook for Beginners is your partner on this voyage, and your success in mastering the art of macros is well within reach. So, step into your kitchen, pick up your food scale, and create the macros to define your healthier, more balanced lifestyle. Bon appétit!

# TABLE OF MEASUREMENT UNITS

| INGREDIENT | CUPS | GRAMS | OUNCES |
|---|---|---|---|
| All-Purpose Flour | 1 cup | 120g | 4.2 oz |
| Whole Wheat Flour | 1 cup | 130g | 4.6 oz |
| Granulated Sugar | 1 cup | 200g | 7.1 oz |
| Brown Sugar | 1 cup | 220g | 7.8 oz |
| Powdered Sugar | 1 cup | 120g | 4.2 oz |
| Butter | 1 cup | 227g | 8 oz |
| Olive Oil | 1 cup | 216g | 7.6 oz |
| Milk | 1 cup | 240g | 8.5 oz |
| Water | 1 cup | 240g | 8.5 oz |
| Honey | 1 cup | 340g | 12 oz |
| Yogurt | 1 cup | 240g | 8.5 oz |
| Rice (uncooked) | 1 cup | 185g | 6.5 oz |
| Pasta (uncooked) | 1 cup | 140g | 4.9 oz |
| Quinoa (uncooked) | 1 cup | 185g | 6.5 oz |
| Lentils (uncooked) | 1 cup | 200g | 7.1 oz |
| Chickpeas (canned) | 1 cup | 240g | 8.5 oz |
| Almonds | 1 cup | 140g | 4.9 oz |
| Walnuts | 1 cup | 125g | 4.4 oz |
| Tomatoes (diced) | 1 cup | 240g | 8.5 oz |
| Cucumbers (sliced) | 1 cup | 119g | 4.2 oz |
| Bell Peppers | 1 cup | 149g | 5.3 oz |

| INGREDIENT | CUPS | GRAMS | OUNCES |
| --- | --- | --- | --- |
| Spinach (fresh) | 1 cup | 30g | 1.1 oz |
| Basil (fresh) | 1 cup | 21g | 0.7 oz |
| Feta Cheese | 1 cup | 150g | 5.3 oz |
| Greek Yogurt | 1 cup | 245g | 8.6 oz |
| Olives (pitted) | 1 cup | 180g | 6.3 oz |
| Honey | 1 cup | 340g | 12 oz |
| Red Wine Vinegar | 1 cup | 240g | 8.5 oz |
| Lemon Juice | 1 cup | 240g | 8.5 oz |
| Balsamic Vinegar | 1 cup | 240g | 8.5 oz |
| Hummus | 1 cup | 240g | 8.5 oz |
| Tahini | 1 cup | 240g | 8.5 oz |
| Greek Salad Dressing | 1 cup | 240g | 8.5 oz |

Limitation of Liability / Disclaimer of Warranty: The publisher and the author of this work are not medical professionals and do not provide medical counseling, treatments, or diagnoses. The contents of this work are provided for informational purposes only and should not be considered a substitute for professional medical advice. The publisher and the author make no warranties or representations regarding the accuracy or completeness of the information presented herein. The information in this work has not been evaluated by the U.S. Food and Drug Administration, and it is not intended to diagnose, treat, cure, or prevent any disease. It is recommended that individuals seek full medical clearance from a licensed physician before initiating any diet or health-related practices. The advice and strategies presented in this work may not be suitable for every individual, and the publisher and the author disclaim any responsibility for any adverse effects or consequences resulting from the use, application, or interpretation of the information provided.

Nutritional Information: The nutritional information provided in this work is based on specific brands, measurements, and ingredients used in the recipes. It is intended for informational purposes only and should not be considered a guarantee of the actual nutritional value of the reader's prepared recipe. The publisher and the author are not responsible for any damages or losses resulting from reliance on the provided nutritional information.